Healthy, West African & Wise™

The Complete Guide to a Healthy West African Diet and Lifestyle

Healthy, West African & Wise™

The Complete Guide to a Healthy West African Diet and Lifestyle

Angela Tella, RD

Illumina Press

This edition first published in the UK in 2010 by
Illumina Press
Petworth Way
RM12

Cover design: Multimedia Styles
Editor: Ben Robertson
Production: S4E Media

A CIP record for this book is available at the British Library.

ISBN 978-0-9566660-0-0

Printed and bound in India by Print Vision.

Publisher's note: The information in this book is intended as general diet and lifestyle advice. No responsibility can be taken by the author for misuse of the information provided, nor does it replace individual dietary advice from a registered dietitian or proper medical diagnosis by a doctor. All information provided was correct at time of print.

Contents

Acknowledgments

This book is the realisation of a dream – one of those dreams that niggle away at you and won't go away till you've done something about it. It takes more than an author to bring any book idea to life and my sincere thanks and appreciation go to everyone who 'hassled' me to put paper to pen and played an integral part in this project.

I especially want to thank my husband and biggest cheerleader, Ben, who has always believed in me and actively encouraged me to follow my dreams. Thanks for all the moral and practical support you gave during this project - here's to many more!! My daughter Zoë, for being so patient and grown up about the fact that I had to write at some of the most inconvenient times. My resourceful parents, Mr & Mrs Uche, for their unwavering support and for giving me a taste of West Africa (specifically Nigeria) early on in life - the experience has proven invaluable. To the entire Illumina Press team, especially Jazmine Emeagi and Sonny Samuel – we actually did it!!! How can I ever thank you?

A big thank you to Sheila Addison, for being a wonderful mentor and Edward Addison, for helping sort through my initial thoughts and ideas, helping channel my restlessness and giving constructive feedback! Special thanks go to Weight Concern for allowing me to use their 'Getting the Balance Right' plate model. Finally, to everyone who knowingly (or unwittingly) helped make this dream a reality: you made the mountain-sized obstacles along the way become mere molehills - thank you!

“Helping others is good; teaching them to help themselves is better.”

George Orwell

Foreword

At last! Clear, practical, guidance on how to make diet and lifestyle changes for healthier living, based on West African foods. These days, many people are looking for ways to make healthy changes in their diet and lifestyle, but amongst all the books, websites and other sources of information, it is sometimes difficult to find advice that is reliable, practical and based on the foods we like to eat – more so if our favourite dishes are based on West African cuisine.

Food is about enjoyment as well as health, and it is hard to enjoy food if it doesn't taste good or contains unfamiliar ingredients - after all, food is part of the glue that holds families and friends together! Most of us are also pressed for time and even when we have good intentions, these can fly out of the window when making quick decisions at the supermarket, or eating out. The practical tips in this book can make life not only healthier, but easier.

This book is long overdue and based on her professional knowledge and personal experience, Angela Tella RD is well qualified to provide this authoritative, practical information that can make change possible for anyone who enjoys West African foods. It will also be an invaluable resource for health professionals, especially dietitians, who want to give advice that people can actually follow and continue to enjoy the pleasures of eating.

Jane Thomas RD FBDA

Senior Lecturer in Nutrition & Dietetics

King's College London

Foreword

Advising the UK government on how best to engage ethnic minority communities to ensure that they are informed about new government initiatives, and more importantly, to encourage behaviour change so as to tackle some of society's most intractable and costly problems, (for example, the rising tide of obesity), is not only challenging but fascinating.

Being of West African descent, I know how important food is in our culture, especially our traditional cuisine. So when I became involved in the UK government's Change4Life initiative to tackle childhood obesity and encourage at-risk groups (West Africans being one them), to make changes to their diets and be more physically active, I knew I had my work cut out.

There is a high prevalence of diabetes, stroke and heart disease (which are all obesity-related diseases), in the West African community. In fact, most West Africans know someone in their family or social circle that suffers from one or more of these diseases. Additionally, many of us are aware that our traditional cuisine, as tasty as it is, has played a major role in the West African community being more susceptible to these diseases - therefore there is no denying that something has to change.

I believe Angela Tella has the answers to help the West African community eat healthier and become more active, whilst still maintaining cultural values. I saw Angela in action when we ran a series of cooking demonstrations in community settings, and I can testify that she really knows her stuff when it comes to diet, nutrition and West African culture. She certainly challenged any misconceptions the audience and I had - that if you make small changes to the recipe of a traditional dish like jollof rice or okra soup, you would compromise on taste. This was far from the truth and we were all pleasantly surprised when it came to tasting the dishes - even the more experienced cooks in our midst were amazed. By making small diet and lifestyle changes as a community, we can ensure that we have positive health outcomes for both ourselves and the next generation of West Africans.

This book is the first of its kind and a must-read for every West African and anyone who enjoys West African cuisine. Among other things, it will provide valuable insight into the West African diet and provide lots of practical tips to help ensure that you, your family and generations to come have healthier lifestyles whilst enjoying traditional West African cuisine.

Patricia Macauley
Head of Cultural Diversity
UK Government Central Office of Information

Introduction

The relationship between health, diet and lifestyle is one that is always of major interest to the public and professionals alike. In line with global trends, the UK has experienced an increase in diet and lifestyle-related diseases, with research showing that Black and Minority Ethnic (BME) communities are more likely to experience poor health due to poor diet and lifestyle. Consequently, there is an increasing awareness amongst UK healthcare providers and relevant government agencies of the need to tackle diet and lifestyle-related health issues within BME communities in culturally appropriate ways that BME communities can understand and identify with. Members of these communities also want to take charge of their health and the West African community is no exception. This book aims to empower the West African community to do just that, by providing relevant information and guidance on how to achieve a healthy diet and lifestyle.

Being of West African origin, I fully understand the frustration of trying to eat healthily without culturally relevant information on the subject. My professional experience as a registered dietitian exposed me to the glaring fact that the healthy eating information available on West African foods was limited; it did not cover the wide range of foods eaten by West Africans and was not always culturally sensitive. This, coupled with never-ending questions from fellow West Africans asking for my opinion on West African foods and healthy eating, is what birthed the concept for this book. Acting as the West African nutrition expert for the UK Department of Health's Change4Life BME national campaign, further highlighted the need for a more comprehensive and yet suitable approach to addressing the diet and lifestyle-related health issues that our community faces.

So here it is. A book designed to speak to you the reader. A book that uniquely addresses your diet and lifestyle needs as a person of West African origin. This book aims to not only explain the healthy eating message, but also to enable you apply it in your everyday life. Though the main focus is diet, the significance of West African culture and other lifestyle factors and how they impact on health is covered too. My intention is to highlight the positive aspects of our diet and lifestyle and also get you thinking about what you can do to change the negatives. Hopefully, the end result of reading this book will be an increased awareness about West African diet, lifestyle and health, as well as a more empowered you - making the right choices and living a healthier life.

This book highlights some of the key health and nutritional benefits of some common West African foods, and provides some traditional West African names. More detailed profiles for over 80 individual foods (with colour photos, fascinating facts, invaluable health and nutritional information, and more West African names), can be found in my accompanying book, the *Healthy, West African and Wise™ Food Guide.*

I firmly believe that it is also very important to get the balance right with non-West African foods that form an integral part of the West African diet, else all our hard work in changing our approach to traditional foods will be undone. To this effect, this book provides information on some Western foods too, and how they can be incorporated into a healthy West African diet.

To get the most out of this book, there are some practical activities aimed at getting you to apply your newly acquired knowledge as you go along. One of the best ways to learn is by doing. Don't worry too much about them; they are simple and straightforward so you should get through them without difficulty. Their purpose is to make what you've learnt clearer and most importantly, to motivate you to put them into practice.

I hope you enjoy reading this book and applying the principles contained in it; I certainly enjoyed writing it. With one turn of this page you'll improve your health and extend your life. So go ahead – start your journey to being Healthy, West African and Wise!

Angela Tella

Chapter 1

So What Are We Doing Wrong?

Recent UK health statistics indicate that as a community, we West Africans are at high risk of developing obesity and, more likely than the UK national average, to suffer type 2 diabetes - a common consequence of obesity. Furthermore, we also experience a significantly high incidence of high blood pressure and therefore stroke. We probably all know of someone who either has one or more of these health conditions or who has lost their life because of them. As sobering as the UK picture is, it is worth pointing out (and worryingly so), that these diet- and lifestyle-related health conditions are also becoming increasingly common in people of West African origin all over the world, including in West African countries. Take for instance the current hot topic of obesity. Figures presented at a recent conference organised by the Oxford Health Alliance suggest that about 35 percent of the Cameroonian population is overweight or obese, with similar rates in the Gambia and Nigeria, particularly among women.

The World Health Organisation estimates that more than 33 percent of African women and 25 percent of African men are overweight, and predicts that this will rise to 41 percent and 30 percent respectively in the next 10 years. These facts all point to one conclusion – we must be doing something wrong. And seeing that these health conditions are diet and lifestyle-related, taking a long, hard look at our diet and lifestyle is a good place to start.

During the early days of my research for this book, I came across a description of West African cuisine as being 'heavy on starch, light on meat and generous in fat'. I whole-heartedly agree with two-thirds of that description: you would have to concur with me that we do have a thing for starchy foods and that oily dishes are (generally) quite the norm for us. I don't quite agree with it being 'light on meat'; from my experience, our cuisine is anything but that. One thing is clear though: many of us have been eating ourselves into poor health and an early grave.

There are several dietary behaviours that are likely to have contributed to the statistics I quoted at the beginning of this chapter. Whilst I don't mean to step on anyone's toes or be controversial, I do hope to provide some food for thought and perhaps challenge some of the things we do as a community. Let's look at our portion sizes for example. As a community we have an 'open house' mentality and a tremendous sense of hospitality – we tend to prepare for unexpected guests by cooking en masse. And in our bid to ensure they are well fed, when they do turn up we dish up large portions. On the receiving end, as guests, hospitality demands that we respond by finishing everything put on our plates and in some instances, politely accepting a second helping - this can program us to eat more than we need. Sometimes we even consciously (or unconsciously) judge a host's levels of hospitality (and status) by how much food and drink is available! Who has never been at a function where the food or drinks ran out and the host was deemed as unable to cater for their guests, or has never heard stories recounted where there was not enough food at a function? With this emphasis on quantity, it's no wonder we are used to large portions.

Some of our cooking practices are not helpful either. We expect certain dishes to taste a certain way because that's how they've always been made to taste. This is understandable for a couple of reasons. Firstly, if that's all we've ever known, our taste buds easily become accustomed to what they are consistently exposed to. Secondly, our food preferences are steeped in West African tradition, reflecting our cultural identity. Unfortunately, our high protein, high fat and high salt dishes are working against us, encouraging weight gain and contributing to our alarmingly high levels of high blood pressure, stroke and diabetes. We will need to challenge our perceptions of taste; would we think differently if we realised that doing things the way they've always been done was negatively affecting our health and shortening our lifespan?

Whilst some of our foods have great health benefits, some of them, due to the amounts we use in our cooking, can have a harmful effect on our health. Considering that we don't usually cook from recipes with measured ingredients, it can be easy to lose track of how much of a particular ingredient we are using. This approach can inevitably result in the generous amounts of oil and more than necessary amounts of salt that we are so accustomed to in our cuisine. Whilst I am not suggesting that we measure absolutely everything, I am saying that in caring for your health it is crucial that you become more aware of how much fat (or oil) and salt you put into your cooking. Too much fat makes you gain weight and if it's saturated fat, it increases your bad cholesterol levels and your risk of heart disease. Likewise, too much salt increases your risk of high blood pressure as well as stroke.

Remember also that your cooking isn't just for you but for other family members, especially your children. Your eating and cooking habits influence your child's dietary behaviour, 'programming' their dietary and taste preferences for life. To put things into perspective, current projections suggest that if we as a community do not change our approach, 9 out of 10 of our children will be obese by 2050. Will your child be one of these?

There also seems to be a particularly prevalent misconception about Western foods in our community. To a large extent we don't regard Western foods as food at all and therefore categorise them as snacks. This is because we perceive them as not being 'substantially filling' or 'heavy' in nature. This belief about these foods means that we tend to discount the calories in them and just like the general population, are not always aware of both the negative (and positive) impact of Western foods on our health.

In addition to dietary behaviours, our attitude towards physical activity possibly hasn't helped either. Due to busyness and other reasons, generally we don't attach much significance to physical activity and are less likely to be involved in physically demanding pursuits in our leisure time than our European counterparts. Similarly, with our children, free time is rather spent on extra tuition or religious education, with little or no room for physical activity. Whilst on the subject of physical activity, for us ladies there is the all-important-and-cannot-be-ignored issue of our hair. Have you ever considered that we have an unspoken rule that says relaxers, perms and weaves don't mix with sweat (and therefore physical activity)?

So now we've looked at what we're doing wrong, let's take a look at how to make things right, as well as answer the burning question, of how the healthy eating message applies to West African food. Many traditional West African foods are naturally full of goodness and low in fat. With just a few simple changes we can enjoy these and many other traditional dishes as part of a healthy balanced diet. Before we do that, carry out the task suggested below.

Activity 1

Keep a record of everything you eat and drink over the next 7 days, including the weekend. Maintain your current eating pattern during this time and don't make any changes. You will need this for the task at the end of the next chapter.

Chapter 2

Healthy Eating, West African Style

Eating healthily is one of the core elements of a healthy lifestyle and is a major focus of this book. A healthy diet enables your body to function well and this in turn makes you feel well. Food provides us with nutrients, and a healthy diet should be a combination of different foods in the right proportions to supply your body with the full range of nutrients it needs to function well. Too little or too much of any nutrient can cause problems, either now or in the future. The nutrients found in food include:

- Carbohydrates, which provide energy;
- Proteins, which are needed for growth and repair of body tissues. These can be from both plant and animal sources;
- Fats, which also provide energy;
- Vitamins and minerals, which though required in smaller amounts, are nonetheless essential to important biochemical processes in the body.

No one particular food contains all the nutrients your body needs and there are no 'good' or 'bad' foods, just healthy or unhealthy diets. Every food you eat contains a combination of these different nutrients but in varying proportions; therefore some foods will be higher in some nutrients than other foods and vice versa. This is why variety is so important. The greater the variety of foods you eat, the more likely your diet will contain all the essential nutrients, especially vitamins and minerals necessary for good health. Variety also ensures that you enjoy eating – having the same thing over and over can get quite boring after a while!

"The healthy eating message sounds brilliant, but how does this apply to *our* food, traditional West African food?" I hear you ask. This is a really pertinent question, especially if you've ever sought advice from experts and been given nutrition information that has been less than helpful. Traditional West African foods are rarely (if at all) represented on healthy eating plans, and so it is easy to believe that our foods can't be part a healthy eating plan.

So, how does the healthy eating message apply to traditional West African foods? The answer to that question lies in putting each food in its rightful place and to do this, let's takes a look at the figure on the next page. It is based on the UK government's guidelines for a healthy diet, and applies to most people except those with special dietary requirements due to certain medical conditions, and children under the age of two.

You'll notice that many of your favourite West African foods have a home in this figure. I would also like to emphasise three key concepts that this 'Getting the Balance Right' model strongly encourages: variety, balance and moderation, all of which we can apply to our individual diets. There are also two important take-home messages. Firstly, it's the overall content of your food intake over a day, week or month that matters and secondly, all foods can fit into a healthy diet as long as they are eaten in the right proportions.

As such, it is also important to come to grips with the concept of portion control, especially within West African culture where large portions tend to be the norm. Research shows that large portions encourage us to eat more – the more you see, the more you eat! A study published in the American Journal of Clinical Nutrition showed that when individuals were given larger portions, they ate more

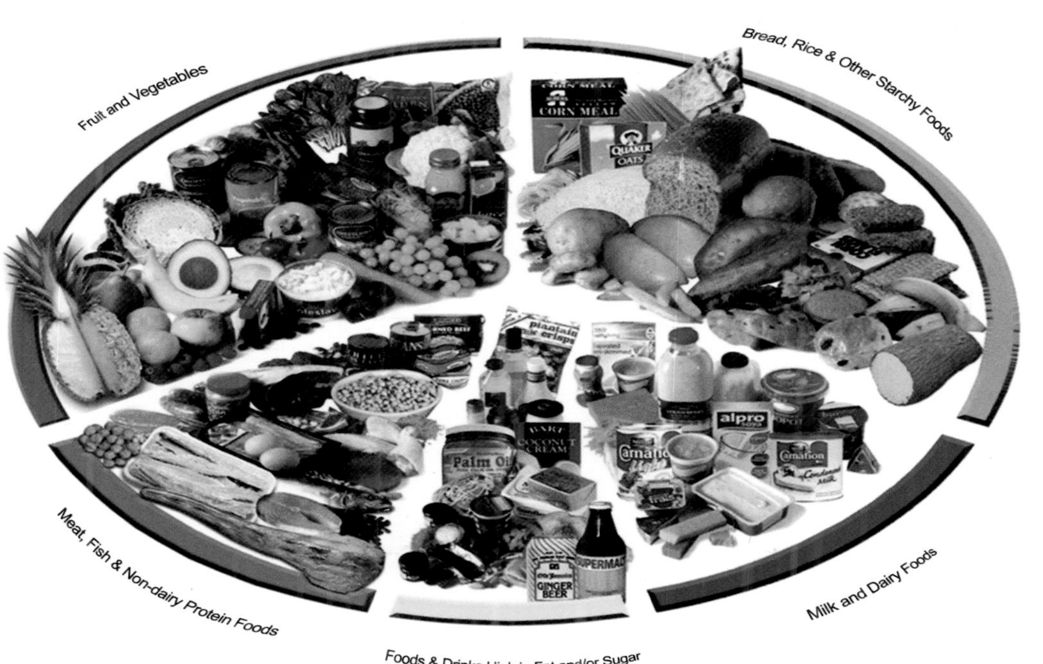

Adapted and used by kind permission of Weight Concern

without feeling any fuller than when given smaller portions. This illustrates how portion size influences the amounts we are able to eat and how easily we can get used to larger portion sizes. Consequently, feeling full is not determined by portion size and you can be just as full with smaller portions as you would with larger portions. Therefore, we need to rid ourselves of the popular approach to food which is to fill every nook and cranny of the stomach.

In the next section, we will look in more detail at the food groups found in the 'Getting the Balance Right' model. This section also provides guidance on serving sizes for each food group. As a portion of food will consist of one or more servings, the serving guides will enable you determine the right amounts to eat.

Bread, Rice and Other Starchy Foods
How much: 6-11 servings daily

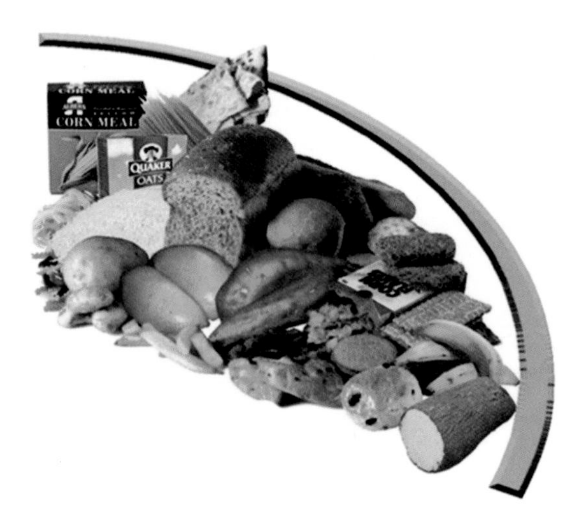

These provide readily available energy or fuel for the body. Once eaten and digested, starchy carbohydrates are converted into glucose, which is then used by the body to meet its energy needs. The benefit of these foods as energy sources is that they are generally digested slowly and the energy in them is released over a period of time, thereby keeping you fuller for longer. They are also sources of other key nutrients including B vitamins, iron, calcium, magnesium and fibre.

Current UK healthy eating guidelines recommend that starchy or complex carbohydrates should form the basis of all meals and, as West African meals are based on starchy foods, our diet is perfectly in line with government recommendations for good health. Contrary to popular belief, these foods are not 'fattening' in themselves. Also, they do not contribute to weight gain except when fats and oils are added to them, or if very large amounts are consumed over a period of time. This is because, like all food, starchy foods contain calories (4 calories per gram), and any calories eaten in excess of what your body needs will be stored as excess weight.

On average, 6 to 7 servings of starchy food per day is sufficient for most people, though this will very much depend on a number of factors including activity levels and gender. The problem starts when we begin to consider that West African meals can contain large amounts of starchy food, so it's no surprise that our intake of these can be excessive, especially when our portion sizes are taken into account! We need to be more aware of our portion sizes and use less fat in preparing these foods as well as other dishes that we serve alongside them. Foods commonly eaten in this group include:

- Starchy roots and tubers such as yam, cassava, sweet potatoes, Irish potatoes and cocoyam. Also their products, including yam flour (*lafun, elubo*), fermented cassava flour (*garri, farina*), dried and fresh shredded cassava (also known as *abacha*), fermented cassava dough (*fufu*), unfermented cassava dough (*dumboy*), steamed, fermented cassava granules (*attieke)*, and cassava flour (*kokonte*).

- Cereals such as rice, millet, fonio, wheat, corn and guinea corn and their products. These include ground rice and *tuwo shinkafa*, corn on the cob, cornmeal, fermented porridges (*ogi, akamu, koko*), fermented corn dough (*tuwo masara, kenkey, mawe, banku*), thick-set fermented porridge (*eko, agidi, akassa*), and couscous.
- Breakfast cereals such as cornflakes, porridge oats, Shreddies, Shredded Wheat, Weetabix, Rice Krispies, Branflakes and muesli.
- Breads of different kinds, such as West African breads (*Agege bread, Ghana bread*), ciabatta, granary, baguette, West Indian hard dough bread, malt bread, wholemeal bread and pitta.
- Starchy fruits such as plantain.
- Starchy seeds such as those of the African breadfruit (also known as *ukwa, afon, brebretim, morkungo*).

Food	**One serving***
Breakfast cereal	3 tablespoons
Weetabix or Shredded Wheat	1 biscuit
Bread	1 slice (as thick as an audio cassette)
Pitta bread	1 mini or ½ large
Pasta/noodles (cooked)	1 heaped handful
Plantain	½ large
Green banana	1 small
Potato (boiled)	1 egg-sized

Food	One serving*
Garri (uncooked)	3 heaped tablespoons or 1 heaped cooking spoon (approx 40g)
Ground rice or pounded yam flour (uncooked)	2 heaped tablespoons or 1 level cooking spoon (approx 40g)
Garri (cooked)	Tennis ball-sized ball (approx 150g i.e. 40g garri + 110ml water)
Kenkey (cooked)	150g
Boiled cassava or cassava *fufu*	120g
Yam (boiled)	1 slice (as thick as a bar of soap)
Sweet potato (boiled)	1 medium or ½ large (115g)
Rice (cooked)	4 heaped tablespoons or 3 level cooking spoons (approx 100g)

Visualise cooked starchy food to be equivalent to the size of your fist or cupped hand.

Healthy hints:

- Watch your portion sizes. As a guide, starchy foods should make up no more than a third of your plate and a little less if you are trying to lose weight – this is discussed later in this chapter and in the section on weight management in Chapter 5).
- Use cooking methods which do not require fat e.g. boiling, grilling, roasting, steaming. If frying cannot be avoided then limit the quantity eaten and use healthier oils such as corn, soya, groundnut (peanut), sunflower and rape-seed oils.
- Drain or skim off excess oil from soups and stews served with starchy foods.
- Choose wholegrain or higher fibre breakfast cereals such as oats, Weetabix, Shredded Wheat and Branflakes, instead of cereals coated with honey, chocolate or sugar. Eating wholegrain foods as part of a healthy diet contributes to your heart health.

- Avoid adding sugar to foods like potatoes and yam when boiling them.
- Choose higher fibre breads i.e. whole meal, granary and brown varieties. If you absolutely can't stand any of these, there are a variety of high fibre white breads that are now available.
- Limit your intake of breads with added sugar or fat e.g. *Ghana bread* and certain West Indian breads.

The Glycaemic Index

The GI or Glycaemic Index is a way of classifying foods according to how quickly or slowly they release glucose into the bloodstream. Each food is given a number between 1 and 100 depending on its effects on blood glucose levels. High GI foods release glucose quickly into the bloodstream while low GI foods release glucose slowly into the bloodstream.

GI rating	Food examples
Low (GI = 55 or less)	*Kenkey*, cocoyam (boiled and mashed), *kenkey* or unripe plantain (with fish, tomato and onion), unripe plantain (boiled or fried), black-eyed beans, fonio, millet, brown beans, cashew nuts, groundnuts, boiled cassava, green banana (boiled or fried), sweet potato (boiled), corn *fufu* (with *ndole* soup).
Medium (GI = 56 to 69)	Cocoyam (boiled), garri, yam, sugar, mango, pineapple, ripe plantain, papaya.
High (GI = 70 or more)	Yam (boiled or roasted), watermelon, ripe plantain (fried).

Lower GI foods are generally preferable than higher GI foods. However, the GI ratings can be a bit confusing, as some foods which are healthy can have a high GI rating and vice versa. Rather than choose starchy foods based solely on their GI rating, also consider their nutritional value and fibre content. This approach will ensure you eat a wide variety of starchy foods. Eating a low GI food as part of a meal can lower the overall GI of that meal. So, for example, a meal of rice and black-eyed beans will have a lower GI than just rice on its own because black-eyed beans have a low GI.

Meat, Fish and Non-dairy Protein Foods

How much: 2 - 3 servings daily

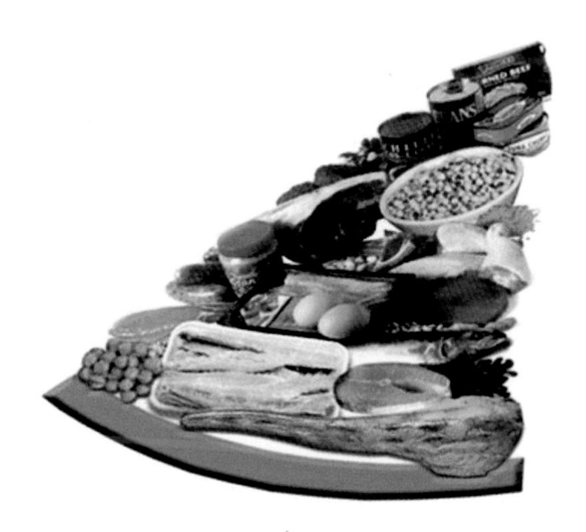

The main role of foods in this group is to provide protein. Protein is used for building and replacing worn-out, wasted or damaged body tissue and is therefore essential for growth. Animal sources tend to provide better quality protein than plant sources but if chosen with care, a dietary intake based on a variety of plant sources can provide enough protein to meet the body's requirements. In addition to providing protein, foods in this group are also sources of minerals like iron, zinc, selenium, phosphorus, magnesium, potassium and iodine, as well as B vitamins. Some foods in this group also provide crucial omega-3 fats. The traditional practice of eating meat off the bone and eating the soft bones of fish and cooked meats means that these foods are also an important source of calcium in the West African diet. Foods in this group include:

- Meats such as beef (including ox-tail), goat, lamb and mutton, pork, and game or 'bush' meats (venison, deer, antelope, rabbit, squirrel, grass-cutter).
- Poultry (fresh or smoked) such as chicken, guinea fowl (*kpwai*), duck and turkey.
- Oily and white fish (fresh, dried or smoked) such as mackerel, salmon, West African herring (*bonga*), West African sardine, barracuda, white-bait, tilapia, croaker (*feta, tonon*), bream, catfish (*koso, okpo, obokun*), red mullet, snapper, tuna, cod (stockfish). Also included are tinned fish products (pilchards, salmon, mackerel and sardines).
- Shellfish such as tropical periwinkles (*isam, kiss meat, abibia),* Man-grove oysters, West African clams (*nkop*), small dried prawns (*crayfish*), large smoked or dried shrimps and prawns (*ede, njanga*), crabs, and crawfish.
- Giant snails (*nwa, kreteke, konk*), considered more of delicacy rather than everyday meats.
- Eggs from chicken, guinea fowl and turkey.

- Nuts and seeds such as dika nuts (*ogbono, apon*), groundnuts (or peanuts), cashews, almonds, walnuts, melon seeds (*egusi*), African oil bean (*ugba, kiriyan, ayan*), tallow tree seeds (*talo, ofo*), African mahogany seeds (*akpalata, konta*), locust beans (*soumbara, dawadawa*), black timber seeds (*tebako, achi*), and African nut tree seeds (*njansang, akpi*).
- Nut butters e.g. peanut butter (plain and spicy).
- Offal such as tripe (*saki, towel, cow goht*), kidney, liver, lungs, gizzard, intestine and tongue.
- Pulses and legumes such as black–eyed beans (*soso, haricot*), soya beans, Bambara beans (*bamoyu, mankara di biago*), African yam beans (*akitereku*), pigeon peas (*kongo binch, feijao Congo*), horse eye beans (*ukpo, osayai binch*) and lima beans (*tubabu soso, kissi soso*).
- Edible insects such as termites (*esunsun, aku*) are considered a delicacy, especially due their seasonal nature.

Though commonly viewed as meat, cow feet (*kaufut*) and cow skin (*pomo, kanda*) should not be classified as meat, due to their nutritional composition (see the accompanying *Healthy West African and Wise™ Food Guide* for more information on this). Likewise, due to their high fat content, pigs' feet and ham hocks have been classified as high fat foods (see the *Foods and Drinks High in Fat and/or Sugar* section in this chapter).

Food	**One serving***
Lean meat (cooked and without bone)	80g or size of a deck of cards or bar of soap
Chicken or guinea fowl	1 thigh, 1 drumstick or similar sized piece
Fish	Small tin or size of deck of cards

Food	One serving*
Tropical periwinkles (shelled)	100g
Giant West African land snails (shelled, and cleaned)	140g
Eggs	2
Nuts	Small handful or 2 tablespoons
Nut products e.g. peanut butter	2 tablespoons
Cooked beans or pulses	3 heaped tablespoons
Soya, tofu or textured vegetable protein e.g. Quorn	40g or small match box size
Baked beans or similar West African bean dishes	5 tablespoons or 1 small can

Visualise a serving of meat to be the size of your palm and as thick as your small finger.

Healthy hints:

- Cool and refrigerate meat stock and dispose of the resulting solid fat layer. This is saturated fat which has been proven to increase cholesterol levels and therefore the risk of heart disease.
- Avoid cheaper cuts of meat which tend to be fatty e.g. mutton; buy lean cuts of meat instead. Remove visible fat if present and take skin off chicken, guinea fowl and turkey.
- Where available, use reduced-fat peanut butter for sandwiches, and smaller amounts of full-fat peanut butter in cooking.
- Fish is a good alternative to meat as it contains less saturated fat. Aim to have at least 2 portions of fish every week, one of which should be oily fish, (a good source of omega-3 fatty acids which are beneficial to heart health). An adult portion is about 140 grams and suitable fish include mackerel, salmon, herring, sardines, and pilchards. More information on omega-3 fats, including plant sources, is provided in the *Foods and Drinks High in Fat and/or Sugar* section in this chapter.

- Girls, as well as women who are breastfeeding, pregnant or of childbearing age, should have a maximum of 2 portions of oily fish per week. Men, boys and women past childbearing age can have up to 4 portions a week.
- Try roasted, unsalted soya beans (soya nuts) as a lower calorie alternative to peanuts, almonds and cashew nuts. In the UK they are widely available in supermarkets.
- Aim to eat no more than 500g of cooked, red meat per week to reduce your risk of colorectal cancer. Also, keep your intake of processed meats (e.g. corned beef, bacon, ham, hot dogs) to the barest minimum, as they are high in salt which can increase your risk of stomach cancer and high blood pressure.
- Offal like heart, liver and kidney are nutritious, lean and low in fat. Liver, for example, is high in iron and vitamins A and D, but limit your intake of this if you are pregnant.
- A portion of pulses, such as beans, can also count towards your vegetable intake. However, regardless of how much you have, it will only count as one portion.

Protein in West African cuisine

West African soups and stews can contain different cuts of meat, poultry, fish and shellfish all in one pot. This practice can however result in unnecessarily high protein intake, especially from meat. Eating too much protein has been associated with osteoporosis and kidney disease, and eating too much red meat has been linked to bowel cancer. Furthermore, we have a tendency to favour poultry with the skin on as well as fatty meats like mutton and lamb. It is therefore important to keep an eye on portion sizes and also be aware of alternative protein sources. These include pulses and legumes, and foods based on them, such as one-pot bean casseroles and stews, bean fritters (*akara, kose*), and steamed bean pudding (*moin-moin, oleleh*).

Fruit and Vegetables

How much: At least 5 servings daily

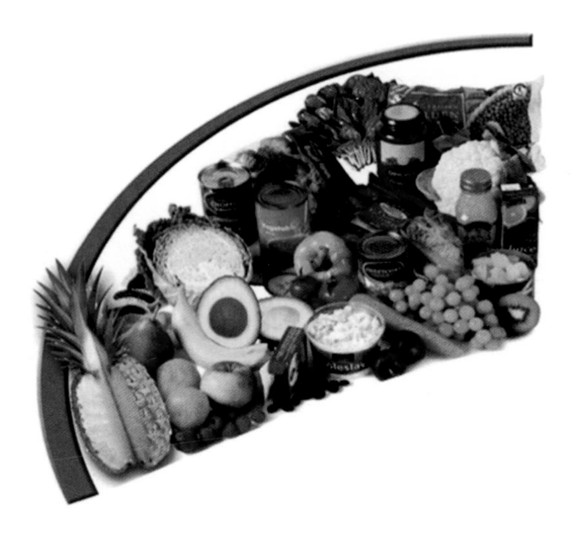

These are very good sources of vitamins C and E, folic acid, beta-carotene, magnesium, potassium, calcium, iron, and both soluble and insoluble fibre. They also contain phytochemicals, which are natural plant compounds that have protective properties. Fruit and vegetables are low in calories, making them excellent and convenient snacks and their high potassium content helps maintain healthy blood pressure levels. Additionally, fresh and dried leafy green vegetables are especially important in the West African diet because they are a major source of calcium which has also been proven to help lower high blood pressure levels. For example, 9g of dried baobab leaves and 47g of cooked African spinach each provide the same amount of calcium as a glass of milk. Commonly eaten fruit and vegetables in the West African diet include:

- Fruit and fruit juices such as guava, mango, pineapple, citrus fruit (orange, grapefruit, lime and lemon), pawpaw (papaya), banana, baobab fruit, watermelon, cashew fruit, pineapple, sugarcane, avocado, velvet tamarind (*ichekwu, solom*), pear, apple, African pear (*safou*), White star apple (*udara, agbalumo*), almond tree fruit, bush mango, gum vine fruit, sour sop, and wild mango.
- Salad and fruit vegetables such as tomato, bell or sweet pepper, scotch bonnet peppers (*ijoko, ata rodo*), bird peppers (*ata, kaani*), cabbage, lettuce, onion, carrot, cucumber, bitter tomato, African eggplants (*bitter balls*), okra (*gombo, kanja*), pumpkin and aubergine.
- Leafy green vegetables such as leaves from the following plants: fluted pumpkin (*ugu, obong*), African joint fir (*okazi, afang*), African spinach (*tete, asibe*), jute (*ewedu, kirinkirin, mbali*), bitter leaf (*ndo*), Lagos spinach (*soko, boh*), waterleaf (*bologi*), African padouk (*oha*), baobab (*kuka, lalo*), red sorrel (*ishapa, sawa*), rag leaf, pumpkin (*ugboguru, elegede*), cassava (*nyambi jambo, nkwem*), sweet potato (*saga saga*), African eggplant, bush apple (*nonohi, kpia-kpia*).
- Mushrooms of various kinds, which are used as meat substitutes in some parts of West Africa.
- Tender shoots of elephant grass (*achara*), which are used in soups and stews in some parts of West Africa.

Fruit and vegetables have validated health benefits and the World Health Organisation recommends a daily intake of at least 400g. This equates to at least five 80g servings daily, which translates into three servings of fruit plus two servings of vegetables. In practical terms, a serving is simply what you can fit into a cupped hand, as illustrated in the serving size guide.

Food		**One serving**
Dried fruit	Raisins	1-1½ tablespoons
Very small fruit	Berries, grapes, cherries, velvet tamarind (peeled)	1 small cup or a handful
Small fruit	Plum, kiwi, tangerine, white star apple	2 fruit
Medium fruit	Apple/banana/orange	1 medium
Large fruit	Papaya , watermelon, pineapple	1 large slice (1 inch thick)
	Mango, avocado, grapefruit	½ fruit
Fruit juice/vegetable juice/100% fruit smoothie		1 small glass (150ml)
Leafy green vegetables (cooked)		3 heaped tablespoons or 1 cooking spoon
Salad vegetables or raw leafy green vegetables		1 large cereal bowlful
Tomatoes		1 medium or 7 cherry tomatoes

Fruit juice can be part of your 5-a-day, but regardless of how much you drink, only one small glass of juice (about 150ml) counts as a portion. You may find it easier to get through your 5 portions on some days but not on others; you may also find that you get through more vegetable portions than fruit, and vice versa. As long as you aim for at least 5 portions, that should suffice. However, do try and aim to have a good mix of fruit and vegetables.

Healthy hints:

- Get into the habit of serving vegetables at every meal as a means of bringing balance to your meal and achieving your 5-a-day target.
- Serve fruit after meals, particularly after soups containing bitter leaf, cassava leaves or sour leaves, to recoup vitamins lost during the prerequisite pounding, washing and bruising of these leaves.
- Make your 5-a-day intake more colourful and interesting by having fruit and vegetables of different colours. Be adventurous and try something you've never had before.
- Eating vegetable-containing soups and stews is a good way of capturing important vitamins and minerals, as long as the vegetables are not overcooked.
- Fruit juice is high in calories so limit your intake, especially if you are overweight. It also does not contain any fibre and should therefore make up only a small part of your daily fruit and vegetable intake. Quench your thirst instead with water (plain, flavoured, or mixed with no-added sugar squash).
- Eat the whole fruit where possible unless the skin is inedible. This ensures that you benefit from the natural fibre in the fruit, as well as the vitamins and minerals. For example, eat the edible parts of an orange rather than just sucking on it.
- Frozen fruit and vegetables are just as good as fresh, dried, tinned or canned versions. Tinned or canned fruit is also great from a convenience point of view. Just make sure the fruit is tinned in juice instead of syrup and choose reduced-salt versions of tinned vegetables where available.

5–A–Day know-how

Despite the variety of fruit available and the growing evidence supporting the benefits of fruit and vegetables, fruit consumption remains low in the UK. Research also shows that compared to other foods, fruit consumption remains low in West Africa from infancy and throughout adulthood. Whether due to fruit being out of season or just a plain dislike of fruit, there is the possibility that this fact also rings true of West African communities outside West Africa, since food habits are handed down through generations and are part of our culture. Five servings a day may sound like a lot but is relatively easy to achieve. It's all about fitting your five servings into your day, so personalise it! Here is an example of how to do this:

- Breakfast with one serving of fruit e.g. a small glass of fruit juice.
- One serving of fruit as a mid–morning snack e.g. a small handful (8-10) of grapes or shelled velvet tamarind.
- Lunch with a serving of fruit and a serving of vegetables e.g. *jollof rice*, a bowl of salad (with a small amount of light dressing), and a medium-sized banana.
- One serving of vegetables with the evening meal. If you are having a traditional soup or stew, just plate up some extra lightly cooked, steamed or micro-waved vegetables, bearing in mind that one cooking spoonful will count as an adult serving.

Alternatively, you could have a serving of fruit after each meal instead. Just find what works for you. If you have a history of diabetes, remember to never have more than one serving of fruit at any time, to prevent high blood sugar levels.

Foods and Drinks High in Fat and/or Sugar

How much: Eat sparingly and occasionally

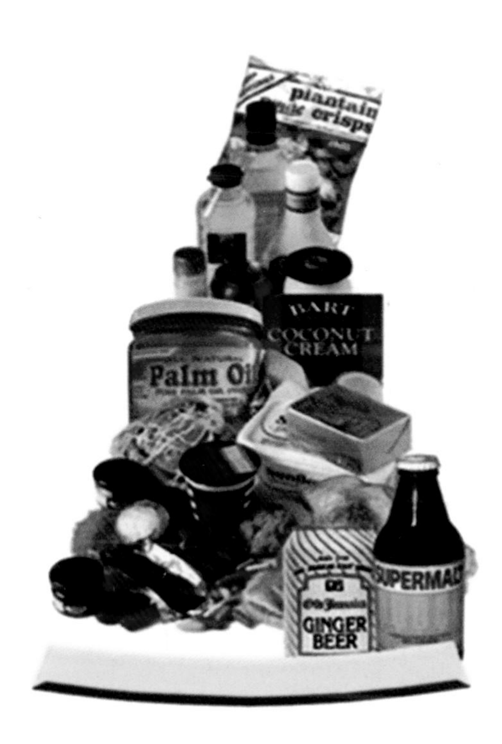

The main role of the foods in this group is to add variety to the diet. Variety, after all, is the spice of life. However, they tend to be high in calories and can contribute to unhealthy weight gain and obesity. There are two main things to be aware of with regard to these foods: the quantity eaten and how often they are eaten.

Rather than being everyday foods, these should be foods that are eaten occasionally. Foods in this group include:

- Snack foods and pastry like fried pastry shapes (*chin-chin*), fried doughnuts (*puff-puff, beignets*), meat kebabs (*suya, chichinga*), bean fritters (*akara, kose*), fried peanut paste shapes (*kuli-kuli, kongu*), fried cornmeal shapes (*kokoro*), meat pies, sausage rolls, cassava chips (*bong fries*), peanut and rice flour candy (*kanya*), *plantain chips*, cocoyam chips (*eddoe*), sweetened and butter popcorn, crisps, cakes and biscuits.
- Beverages such as soft drinks (e.g. Coca Cola, Africola, Limca, Fanta, D'jino and Mirinda), energy drinks (e.g. Lucozade), and malt drinks (e.g. Maltina, Supermalt, Power Malt, Malta Guinness). Also, other sugar-containing beverages like Bournvita, Ovaltine, Horlicks and Milo, as well as traditional homemade drinks made from ginger, hibiscus (*bissap*) or tamarind.
- Sugar and glucose powder.
- Spreads such as margarine, butter, jam, marmalade, mayonnaise and honey.
- Cooking oils and fats such as palm oil and palm (fruit) butter, fermented palm oil (*torbogee oil*), palm kernel oil, vegetable oils, groundnut oil, coconut cream and coconut oil, sesame oil, shea nut oil and butter (*nkuto, ori*), fulla butter or ghee (*sirme, nabam sirme*).
- Sweets, including various traditional West African homemade candies made with peanuts, with coconut and with milk. Also, chocolate and ice-cream.
- Full-fat salad dressings.

- Extra-fatty meats like pigs' feet (*prakontwere*, *ese elede*), and ham hocks. (Even though they are traditionally used as meat, these are high in fat, especially saturated fat. As such, they are high in calories and so are classified as a high fat food to be eaten occasionally).

Unlike other nutrients which have added health benefits attached to their calories, sugar has no nutritional value whatsoever and so provides 'empty calories'. In spite of this, sugar can have a place in a healthy eating plan if eaten in small amounts. Be mindful though that too much sugar can also contribute to tooth decay and poor dental health.

All fats are a concentrated source of calories (one gram of fat provides 9 calories), but some of them do have health benefits. As part of your healthy eating plan you should not avoid fats entirely but aim to have a low fat intake. Here are a couple of reasons for this. Firstly, your body needs some fat to function. For example, certain fats which the body cannot make are a vital component of cells and need to be supplied by what you eat. Dietary fats also provide the fat-soluble vitamins A, D, E and K, and enable your body to absorb them. The second reason is that a fat-free intake is downright awful! Fat adds flavour to food and makes it more palatable - remember healthy eating is also about you enjoying your food.

Keeping an eye on your fat intake

There are two watchwords when dealing with fat – **quantity** and **quality**. Controlling the amount or quantity of fat you use will help to reduce the number of calories from fat in your diet. In addition, paying attention to the type or quality of fat you use is just as important, as it can affect your blood cholesterol levels.

Some of our preferred cooking methods which involve the use of fat or oil, result in high-fat stews, soups and other one-pot dishes. Becoming conscious of the amount and quality of the fat you eat will not only result in reducing your calorie intake, but will also help to keep your heart healthy.

Food	**One serving***
Butter/margarine/spread	1 tea spoon
Reduced-fat margarine or spread	2 teaspoons
Cooking oils (including palm oil)	1 tea spoon
Mayonnaise/salad cream	1 tea spoon
Reduced-fat mayonnaise	2 tea spoons
Crisps, pretzels	1 small bag (25g) , cupped handful
Chocolate	1 small (fun size) bar or ½ regular bar
Chin-chin	1 handful
Plantain chips	30g or ½ packet
Ice cream	1 scoop
Jam/honey	1 heaped tea spoon

For teaspoon measures, visualise a serving as equivalent to the size of the tip of your thumb (i.e. from the tip up to the knuckle).

Healthy hints:

- Use household measures such as cooking spoons, to increase awareness of the amounts of fats and oils you use in cooking.
- Use an artificial sweetener instead of sugar, in homemade sugary drinks and baking. Artificial sweeteners can be even used when to sweeten *garri* steeped in water – and yes, they are safe.
- Watch your consumption of sugar-containing beverages such as Milo, Horlicks and Bournvita. Opt for plain drinking chocolate or cocoa powder

(which does not contain sugar), and if necessary sweeten with artificial sweetener.

- Sports drinks (e.g. Lucozade), malt drinks and ordinary soft drinks are very sugary and therefore high in calories. Aim not to have them often and watch how much you have. A better alternative is to choose sugar-free versions where possible, for example, low calorie or diet soft drinks. You could also split your malt drink into two and top up with diet cola, and lose half the calories in the process.
- Snacks such as chin-chin, plantain chips, and puff-puff are high in calories and should be eaten infrequently and in small quantities.
- Use light or reduced-fat coconut milk to cook coconut rice, instead of coconut cream or full-fat coconut milk.
- Reduced-fat salad dressings can be just as tasty as full-fat ones. Nevertheless, pay attention to how much you use as they still contain fat and therefore calories.
- Limit how much and how often you eat high-fat dishes such as palm fruit (*palm butter*) soup and high-fat foods such as pigs' feet.
- Honey, though natural, contains 'empty' calories just like sugar – it has little, if any, nutritional value. Similarly, 'light or half-spoon' sugars contain 50 percent sugar and are therefore still a source of 'empty' calories.
- Brown sugars such as demerara or muscovado are no different in nutrient and calorie content compared to white sugar. The only difference is the extent to which they have been processed or had their natural colouring removed. The darker the sugar, the less processing it has been subjected to.

Omega-3: A good fat

Omega-3 fats are a type of polyunsaturated fat and are present in some plants and fish. In plants, they are found as alpha linoleic acid (ALA); in fish they are found as docosahexanoic acid (DHA) and eicosapentanoic acid (EPA). Studies of populations that eat fish regularly, such as the Japanese and Eskimos, show that there is a relationship between their regular fish intake and their lower rate of heart disease. Omega-3 fats may therefore help to improve heart health by:

- Helping to control blood pressure.
- Reducing the stickiness of the blood, therefore reducing the likelihood of blood clot formation.
- Regulating heart beat and improving the elasticity of arteries.
- Reducing triglyceride (a type of fat) levels in the blood. High levels are associated with increased risk of heart disease.
- Reducing the furring up process in the arteries.

Additionally, omega-3 fats are important for the healthy development of the brain and eyes in unborn babies. Recent studies also suggest that they may enhance children's learning and concentration, and their anti-inflammatory properties may help to reduce joint stiffness.

Oily fish is the better source of omega-3 fats. However, if you do not eat fish, plant sources are better than none at all. The recommended intake of omega-3 is 450mg/day. In practical terms, this translates to 2 portions of oily fish per week and a portion is about 140g (5oz). Good sources of omega-3 fats in the West African diet include dark green leafy vegetables, soya beans, bonga fish and mackerel. More sources can be found on the next page.

Fats are made of building blocks called fatty acids. All foods contain a mixture of the different fatty acids but in different proportions, and are classified according to the largest proportion of fatty acids they contain. The table below shows the different fatty acids found in food, their sources in the West African diet, as well as their effects on levels of High Density Lipoprotein and Low Density Lipoprotein cholesterol i.e. good and bad cholesterol respectively:

Fat		Comments	Dietary Sources	Effects on blood cholesterol
Monounsaturated Fatty Acids (MUFA)		Best type of fat.	Olive oil, avocados, groundnut oil, rapeseed oil[1], tiger nuts, African pear.	Raises 'good' and lowers 'bad'.
Polyunsaturated Fatty Acids (PUFA)	Omega-3	Second best type of fat. Cannot be made by the body therefore known as essential fatty acids.	Walnuts, oily fish like sardines, salmon, pilchards, West African herring (*bonga fish*), mackerel, tuna (fresh or frozen only); soya beans, soya milk and soya oil, *crayfish*, mangrove oysters, tropical periwinkles.	Minimal effects on blood cholesterol.
	Omega-6		Sunflower, safflower, corn and soya oils. Also oils found in melon seeds (*egusi*) and dika nuts (*ogbono*), African oil beans, tiger nuts, African pear.	Lowers 'bad' but in large amounts can also lower 'good'.
Saturated Fatty Acids (SAFA)		Worst type of fat.	Fatty meat, butter, cheese, milk, cream, poultry skin, Coconut cream/oil, palm butter, *torbogee* oil, palm kernel oil and palm oil.	Raises 'bad' and lowers 'good'.

[1] Most oils labelled 'vegetable oil' sold in supermarkets is rapeseed oil, but check the label. Rapeseed oil is a cheaper but just as effective alternative to olive oil.

Fat	Comments	Dietary Sources	Effects on blood cholesterol
Trans Fatty Acids (TFA)[2] or Hydrogenated Fat	Similar effects as SAFA.	Commercially manufactured foods like cakes, biscuits, pies and vegetable oils heated repeatedly.	Raises 'bad' and lowers 'good'.
Dietary Cholesterol	Present in some foods.	Offal such as liver, kidney, tripe and intestine, egg yolks and shellfish such as prawns, shrimps, crab and lobster.	Negligible unless eaten in very large quantities.

[2] Trans fatty acids are formed when vegetable oils are artificially hardened. They are also created naturally in the stomachs of sheep and cows and therefore are found in small quantities in animal products (milk, cheese, lamb and beef). Some research suggests that these natural trans fats can actually have a beneficial effect on cardiovascular disease, diabetes and immune response.

Milk and Dairy Foods

How much: 2-3 servings daily

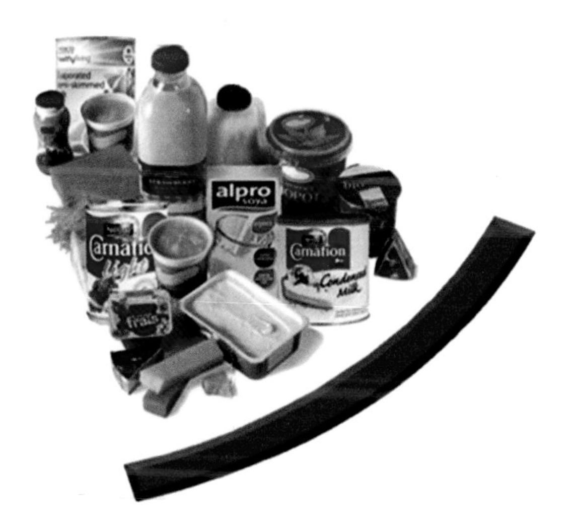

Foods in this group are excellent sources of protein, calcium and the fat-soluble vitamins A and D. The downside is that they can be high in calories if they are full-fat versions or, in the case of sweetened condensed milk, high in sugar. Traditionally, fresh milk and dairy products are not eaten in large quantities in West African countries, and when they are, they tend to be eaten mainly amongst nomadic, pastoralist tribes. Historically, this was because rearing cattle was made difficult by the presence of the *tsetse fly*, which caused disease amongst cattle in the coastal areas of West Africa. Incidentally, research shows that people of African origin are less likely to suffer from bone fractures or osteoporosis (thinning of the bones partly caused by a lack of calcium), than people of other races. This suggests that despite the relatively small amounts of dairy foods we eat, we must be meeting our calcium requirements from other food sources. Additionally, the traditional practice of eating soft bones in cooked meat, poultry or fish (including tinned or dried fish), also helps provide calcium - even just eating cooked meat off the bone helps get some calcium in!

Dried milk powder (usually full fat) is more common in West Africa than fresh milk. Evaporated milk and condensed milk are also very popular. The use of these types of milk goes back to colonial days, and amongst West Africans in the UK and around the world, some of these practices continue because they were handed down through the generations. The main dairy products used by West Africans include:

- Milk including full-fat, semi-skimmed and skimmed varieties (fresh and powdered), and sweetened and unsweetened condensed and evaporated milk.
- Yoghurt and yogurt drinks in full-fat, low-fat and diet varieties, traditional West African yoghurts, and fermented milk drinks such as *nono, kaddam* (*kossam kaddam*).
- Cheeses including European cheeses and West African soft cheese (*wara, warankasi, wagashi* or *wogachi* and *wagassiro*).

Food	**One serving**
Fresh milk	200ml
Calcium-enriched soya milk	200ml
Yoghurt/fromage frais/soft cheese (including traditional West African soft cheeses)	150g or 1 small pot
Skimmed milk powder	20g (2½ tablespoons)
Evaporated milk	85ml (approx 6 tablespoons)
Hard cheese	40g or the size of two 9 volt batteries

Healthy hints:

- Choose low-fat dairy products such as skimmed or semi-skimmed milk. If your taste buds have trouble adapting, try a 50:50 mix of full-fat and semi-skimmed milk and gradually decrease the amount of full-fat milk while increasing the amount of semi-skimmed milk.
- Traditional West African soft cheeses and yoghurts will be high in saturated fat as they are made from full-fat milk, so eat these in small quantities.
- Skimmed and semi-skimmed milks contain more calcium than an equivalent volume of full fat milk - another good reason to use lower fat milks.
- If using dried milk powder, make sure that it is skimmed or semi-skimmed milk and not full fat milk, as is the case of some brands popular amongst West Africans.
- Only use sweetened condensed milk very occasionally, as it is high in calories due to its high sugar content. Evaporated milk can be used more frequently provided you are not overweight or have high cholesterol or triglyceride levels. Alternatively, choose 'light' or low-fat versions.

Lactose Intolerance

Lactose intolerance is common in people of African descent (especially West Africans), and is the most likely reason for the generally relatively low milk and dairy consumption in West African communities. It is caused by low levels of lactase, the enzyme needed to digest lactose, a natural sugar present in milk. In infancy, lactase is present in sufficient numbers but decreases in adulthood. One of the main symptoms of lactose intolerance is wind or flatulence following consumption of a dairy-containing meal. It is not a life-threatening condition.

If you are diagnosed with lactose intolerance it does not mean you have to avoid milk and dairy products. You may find that fermented products such as cheese and yoghurt are better tolerated than milk as they contain little or no levels of lactose. Eat what you can depending on your tolerance and ensure you get the rest of your calcium requirements from other foods (See the quick reference guide for nutrients in Appendix 1).

Alternatively, you can choose from the many milk-substitutes that are available on the market – these include soya, oat and rice milks. Just make sure the product you choose has added calcium as some brands do not. There are also reduced-lactose cow's milks i.e. cow's milk with the lactose removed using a special process. Though not 100% lactose-free, the much lower lactose levels make it more suitable for people with lactose intolerance. Goat's milk also contains less lactose than cow's milk.

Last but not least: Fluid

UK government guidelines for healthy eating recommend an average intake of 6 to 8 glasses of fluid daily. This is to prevent dehydration and replace losses of fluid which occur during normal bodily processes of sweating, excretion and breathing. Often, this guideline is misunderstood to mean 6 to 8 glasses of water only or in addition to other drinks taken through the day. Actually, fluids such as water, fruit juices, milk, tea and coffee can all count as part of your fluid intake. However, avoid having too many sugary, fizzy drinks and 100% fruit juices, as they can be high in sugar and therefore calories, resulting in weight gain and dental problems.

In hot weather or during periods of increased activity, fluid losses will be greater and therefore you will need to increase your intake. Having regular drinks through the day is a simple way of ensuring that you get enough fluid. Don't wait till you feel thirsty; oftentimes by the time you feel thirsty you are probably already mildly dehydrated. A quick and easy way of checking if you are drinking enough is to check the colour your urine - pale, straw coloured urine is a good sign, anything darker means you need to drink more.

Bringing balance to your plate

So far we've looked at the three keys to healthy eating (balance, variety and moderation) and we've seen how this applies to what we eat generally. You also now know what constitutes a food serving and how many servings you should aim to have each day. But how do these apply to your plate at mealtimes? As West Africans, our natural affinity for starchy foods means that our meals have a tendency to be quite high in complex carbohydrates with little or no vegetables, and generous helpings of meat, fish and alternatives. As such our plates end up looking like Plate models A and B.

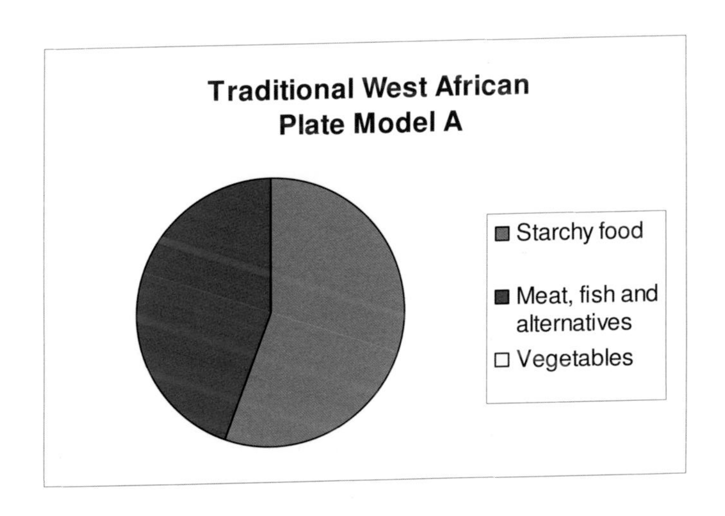

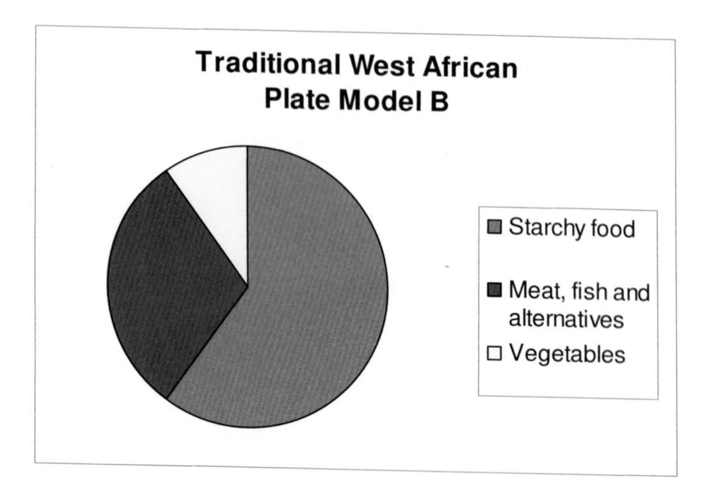

As I pointed out earlier, carbohydrates are not bad; it's just that too much of any food (no matter how healthy), is really excess calories waiting to become excess weight on your waistline. An easy way to achieve balance and manage your portion size at the same time is to be more aware of the amounts of each food group you put on your plate. So in addition to serving sizes, here's another way of getting the balance right at each meal. As a rule of thumb, visually split your plate into 3 equal parts. Fill a third with salad or vegetables and another third with starchy food. Where dairy foods are part of the meal, the final third should be half protein food and half dairy food. For traditional West African meals consisting of a starchy food and a soup or stew, a third of your plate should be starchy food as before, one half of your plate should be vegetables, and what's left (one sixth), your protein source – as in Plate model 1. Most likely, your protein source will be part of the stew or soup, so ensure you have plenty of vegetables (either in the soup or stew or as a side dish), and watch how much oil you use to cook your soup or stew.

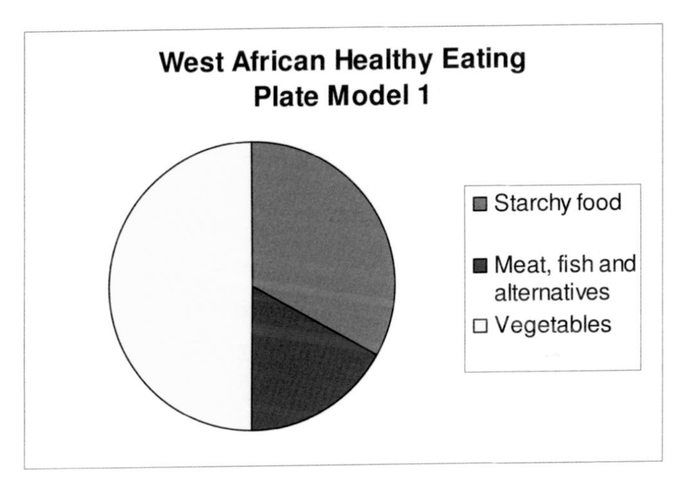

Alternatively, visually divide your plate in two. Fill one half with vegetables or salad. Split the other half into two quarters, one for starchy foods and the other for meat, fish and alternatives, as in Plate model 2. Once again remember to watch how much oil goes into your soup or stew.

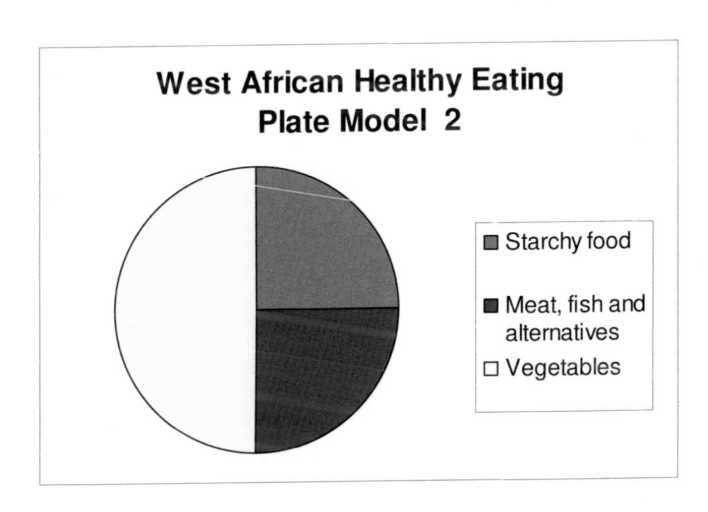

Without much effort, this approach to mealtimes promotes balance, easily overcoming the tendency of typical West African meals to be heavy on starch. It is particularly useful for maintaining a healthy weight, a pre-requisite for good health.

Activity 2

So, if you've ever bought into the idea that West African foods can't be part of a healthy eating plan, I hope I've managed to change your mind. You now know how to classify different West African foods and how many portions you should aim to have daily. Take an honest look at your food diary (which was the suggested activity in Chapter 1) and consider these questions:

- Do you eat regularly and is there a pattern to your eating habits?
- Does your overall daily intake reflect the proportions shown on the 'Getting the Balance Right' model?
- What does your plate look like at mealtimes? What about your portion sizes?
- What are your eating habits like at weekends and during week days? Are they different?

In addition, are you drinking enough through the day to prevent dehydration? You should now be able to identify what necessary adjustments need to be made based on your answers. If you were unable to keep the diary, it is worth doing so now, as it will help increase your awareness of which areas you need to deal with. Identifying a problem is half the problem solved. Your long-term dietary goal is to, as much as possible, make your overall intake reflect the guidelines given by the 'Getting the Balance Right' model, while eating regular meals and keeping an eye on portion sizes. See Chapter 4 on how to set realistic goals and achieve successful and lasting change.

Chapter 3

Don't Worry, Be Happy – And Active

Studies focusing on exercise in our African-American cousins indicate that black people are likely to be less active than their white counterparts. In fact, one study in particular found that those surveyed felt that working out only added stress to their already stressful and hectic lives and that they'd rather relax in their leisure time. Not surprisingly, the research in the UK paints a very similar picture. It is well known that activity levels in Black and Minority Ethnic (BME) communities are lower than for the general population and this was confirmed recently by qualitative research carried out by the UK Department of Health in 2008. The findings show that physical activity levels are low in the West African community, particularly amongst women and children.

Current UK government recommendations are that adults should aim for a minimum of 30 minutes of moderate intensity physical activity daily, on at least 5 days of the week to benefit health. Numerous studies have proven again and again that engaging in regular physical activity can:

- **Reduce your risk of chronic (life-long) health conditions** including diabetes, heart disease, stroke and cancer, as well as improve the management of these conditions. One of the ways physical activity does this is by strengthening your immune system.

- **Help maintain a healthy weight and prevent being overweight.** Physical activity 'burns' excess calories and helps to build lean body tissue or muscle. Your body 'spends' around 20 times more calories to look after muscle tissue than to look after an equal amount of body fat.
- **Improve your sleep pattern.**
- **Help in the management of painful conditions** such as back pain, and leg pain.
- **Help you relax** by combating stress and also increase your energy levels over time.
- **Keep you mentally alert** by aiding more restful sleep, promoting improved concentration and more efficient brain function.
- **Improve your mood.** During physical activity, the brain releases increased amounts of certain chemicals such as dopamine, serotonin and endorphins which have a similar effect as anti-depressants. In fact, in the 1960s and 70s, vigorous walking was used as part of the treatment for depression and anxiety. These chemicals affect a number of body functions including sleep and waking patterns, appetite and even mood.
- **Improve your libido (sex drive).** In addition, your self-esteem and confidence levels can also be given a boost by physical activity.
- **Lengthen your life.** According to a recent study, people over fifty years of age who exercise regularly can live up to four years longer than those who don't.

The evidence above is hard to argue with. So, given the benefits of physical activity, what's stopping us as a community from tapping into the health advantages that physical activity provides?

Why do we have low physical activity levels?

There are many reasons why we have such low physical activity levels and generally don't prioritise exercise – and quite a few of them are valid. We are busy with work, career, family commitments and other responsibilities and, with only 24 hours in any one day, how on earth are we supposed to fit exercise into our already busy lives? Additionally, we may also shy away from exercise because of lack of motivation as well as the financial costs involved, whether actual or perceived. I might add that the weather being too hot or too cold can also get in the way. Then there is the (unspoken) issue in our community of sedentary behaviour being perceived as a status symbol, even more so following retirement. This is especially ironic given our increased risk of developing obesity, diabetes, hypertension and stroke, all of which are proven to be associated with a sedentary lifestyle and increasing age.

For us ladies, even how we wear our hair - coloured, relaxed, permed or in braids or a weave - can get in the way, and there is robust evidence to show that it does. Culturally, our hair is our crowning glory so we go to great lengths to ensure that it looks the part. Consequently, we end up questioning the logic in spending a good chunk of time (and a similar proportion of money) on an amazing hairdo, only to ruin it by deliberately breaking out into a sweat. I'm all for a show-stopping hairstyle but the evidence as regards our health highlights the fact that we need to re-think our stance in letting our hair be a barrier to being physically active.

Overcoming the barriers

So how can we overcome some of the things that are getting in the way of increasing our activity levels? Firstly, I think we need to address the main barrier to being physically active, which is our misconception of what it is all about in the first place. What springs to mind when you hear or think of the word 'exercise'? For most people the word conjures up the image of a gym, complete with fitness fanatics using gym equipment. Or worse, it may bring back really unpleasant memories of being made to participate in school sports against your will (and in some cases, your coach's better judgement). If you've ever thought you could never be 'into' exercise, let me gently remind you that you are highly likely to be already doing some form of exercise on a daily basis. Whether or not you are doing enough is another matter entirely and we'll discuss this later. First of all, let's dispel a couple of physical activity myths.

Myth #1: Being physically active requires going to the gym.

Being physically active does not necessarily call for going to the gym. Most people equate being physically active with going to the gym or taking part in some form of structured activity. Did you know that you can be just as active by not going to the gym? Going to the gym is only one option and is really a question of preference. Bear in mind that having a gym membership and regularly attending the gym are two very distinct things! I hope to get across the life-changing and very liberating message that structured (gym-based) physical activity and lifestyle physical activity are both valid, with the latter being the more realistic option for the majority of people.

Going to the gym may not be for everyone, but it does work. For some, the discipline of the gym keeps them attending. The fact that you've paid for a membership can really sharpen your commitment. It's also an easy way of 'protecting' that time for physical activity and nothing else. For the gym-shy, many different everyday activities can classify as 'exercise' or physical activity. I personally prefer the term 'active living' because it conjures up the idea of making physical activity a part of your daily life and, is less likely to induce a guilt trip. For some people, the thought of going to the gym makes them want to do cartwheels whilst for others it causes them to break out into a cold sweat! If you fall into the latter group (and most people do), then hopefully you'll find some helpful tips in this book.

Myth #2: Exercise is for fitness fanatics and people trying to lose weight.

Being physically active is not just for people trying to lose weight – it's for everyone. Not having any outward signs of ill health does not mean that you are healthy. Believe it or not, slim people can be unhealthy too, so being on the slender side should not be an excuse for not keeping active. To buttress the point, it is possible to be slim and yet have high cholesterol levels that can increase your risk of having a heart attack - I've had clients who were slim yet had either high cholesterol levels or had survived a heart attack.

Practical tips to overcome barriers to physical activity

Even though there may be many barriers to being physically active, my approach has always been to find a way around them because there is always a way. Just because you haven't found a solution doesn't mean that it doesn't exist! Here are some solutions to overcome the main barriers to being physically active – take your pick!

Barrier #1: Lack of Time

This is the barrier that most people use as an excuse to not be active. And while I do agree with the fact that we are busier now than we've ever been, I need to point out that carving time out to be physically active will help you cope with 'busyness' even better. A big chunk of our 'busyness' revolves around school and work, two very important facets of West African life, which I am sure you will agree, would definitely benefit from improved concentration and more efficient brain function – two scientifically proven advantages of physical activity.

Building activity into your daily routine is the best way to overcome this barrier. We each have 24-hours in a day, and what we pack into our 24-hour suitcase will differ from individual to individual, so work out how best to fit active living into your day. Monitor your daily activities for one week and point out at least three 30-minute time slots you could use for physical activity. You then can plan, diarise and protect that time for physical activity and nothing else.

Thirty minutes a day, on at least 5 days a week translates to 2½ hours out of the 168 hours in a week. That is approximately 1.5% of your time over the course of a week! What's more, if 30 minutes at a stretch seems to be a long time, you can spread your 30 minutes over the day e.g. three 10-minute sessions. Flexibility is the name of the game.

Examples of how to build activity into your day include walking or riding your bicycle to work, walking the dog, exercising while you watch TV (one of my favourites), fitting physical activity into your lunch break, and parking further away from your workplace, supermarket or place of worship.

If travel (for business or pleasure) is a regular feature in your life, don't let it get in the way of being physically active. You can pack a skipping rope or resistance band in your suitcase and skip or do some resistance exercises in your hotel room. Choose to walk down corridors and climb the stairs in hotels. Make reservations at hotels that have swimming pools or exercise facilities and pack your mp3 player so you can dance or exercise to your favourite music. If you do go shopping whilst on holiday, visit the local shopping mall and walk for half an hour or more.

Barrier #2: Family commitments

If family commitments, such as caring for children, get in the way, then include the kids! You can spend time together and still get your exercise. Go for a walk together, play tag or other running games. Dance to your favourite fast music or get an aerobic DVD for kids and exercise together. Your children will get into the habit of being physically active and reap the benefits too.

Alternatively, if you want a bit of 'quiet or me time', then consider trading babysitting time with a friend, neighbour, or family member who also has young children. You could also exercise when the kids are not around (for example during school hours or their nap time). You can skip, do calisthenics, ride an exercise bike, or use other home gymnasium equipment while the kids are busy playing or sleeping. I like to put in my exercise just before I go to bed.

Barrier #3: Lack of motivation

If not being motivated enough to start is stopping you from engaging in physical activity, then consider which benefit of being physically active resonates with you – is it better health, improved concentration, better mood or maintaining a healthy weight, or all of them?

Exercising with a friend or an exercise buddy can help keep you motivated as can joining an exercise class or group. Consciously make physical activity a regular part of your daily or weekly schedule by planning ahead and writing it on your calendar. Whatever it is you do, make sure that you are doing something that you enjoy as this will motivate you to do it regularly. If you find your current regime boring then change it - it is extremely rare to need to cajole someone into doing something they actually enjoy!

Barrier #4: Lack of confidence, skill or energy

Focusing on activities that require no new skills, such as walking, climbing stairs, or jogging, can help overcome a lack of confidence. Or, be adventurous and take an exercise class to develop new skills. If being too tired prevents you from being physically active, then plan physical activity for times in the day or week when you feel energetic. Remind yourself that being physically active will increase your energy levels and stamina, and persist with whatever activity you choose to do.

Barrier #5: Cost

There are inexpensive ways of keeping physically fit that cost little or nothing and require minimal facilities or equipment. Never under-estimate the impact that 'free' activities such as walking, jogging or skipping can have on your health and wellbeing. It is also worth looking into physical activity programmes offered by local authorities and community groups, as well as free or discounted work-based exercise programmes and gyms provided by your employer.

Barrier #6: Weather

The easiest way to overcome this barrier is to have a set of regular activities that you can do regardless of the weather – active indoor games, indoor cycling, aerobics, indoor swimming, stair climbing, skipping, mall walking, dancing etc. Home gym equipment and fitness computer games can be used whatever the weather.

Barrier #7: Retirement

Sedentary behaviour is often adopted particularly following retirement. Consciously making the effort to avoid being sedentary is the first step to overcoming this barrier. Start by changing your mindset towards retirement - look at retirement as an opportunity to become more active instead of less. With more time on your hands, plan to make regular physical activity a part of your daily routine. Go for a walk every morning or every evening before dinner. Perhaps get an indoor exercise bike and ride every day while reading a favourite book or magazine. Simple things like getting up to change the TV channel rather than using the remote and limiting screen time - time spent in front of computers and TV – can also make a difference. Playing with grandchildren is another excellent way of keeping fit – it has been said that children with short legs and grandparents with slower gaits are often great walking partners.

Barrier #8: Hair

Neat and stylish hair shows a positive self attitude and makes you feel good about the way you look. If hair concerns are keeping you from exercising, here are a few general tips to protect your hair. You can be fit and keep a beautiful hairstyle too, by protecting your hair and keeping it healthy:

- Wash your hair with a mild, pH-balanced shampoo at least once each week to remove salt build-up from sweat.
- Condition your hair with a moisturising conditioner each time you wash it.
- Avoid over-processing and limit your use of blow dryers and curling irons.
- Pull your hair away from your face and neck when you work out.
- Leave part of your hair unwrapped to breathe whilst working out.
- Get regular cuts or trims to maintain the shape of your hairstyle.

- Ask your hairdresser for help to choose the right hair care products.
- Apply natural oil to your scalp as needed.
- Plan vigorous and longer bouts of physical activity nearer the time of your salon visits.

More hair care tips can be found in Appendix 2.

First steps to becoming more active

If you're seriously considering making that transition from couch potato to being fit and healthy, then start by simply doing more than you currently do. Walking is a great way of increasing your activity levels as it is fundamental to all our daily activities. What's more, it's free and has many benefits, including improving your cardiovascular health, lowering blood pressure and cholesterol levels, and strengthening bones.

Walking is also an easy way to get the benefits of physical activity without creating hair problems that can occur with vigorous or moderate exercise like swimming or cycling. You can easily accumulate your 150 minutes a week in short bouts to prevent perspiration problems.

A good place to start is to assess how much walking you currently do. You can check the number of steps you make already by buying a pedometer. It does not have to be anything expensive as long as it can record your steps. Pedometers have been found to be an effective tool for increasing daily physical activity. They can help you track your progress by providing immediate feedback on your activity levels, and a pedometer attached to your waistband is also a good reminder to be active. Current evidence points to the health benefits associated with taking 10,000 steps a day but this may not be a realistic goal for some. A more realistic approach is to continuously improve on your personal best, and in the process possibly achieving the recommended daily target of 10,000 steps.

No matter what activity you decide on, always think FITT (Frequency = at least 5 days a week; Intensity = moderate; Type = type of activity; and Time = 30 minutes). Moderate intensity activity produces deeper breathing and an increased heart rate. However, you should be able to simultaneously hold a conversation without struggling to do so.

Always speak with your doctor if you have any health conditions or have been inactive for a long period of time before you increase your activity levels. As much as it is important to become active, it is also important that it is done in a way so as not to compromise your health.

And finally...

Encouragingly, the UK Department of Health's research also shows that there does seem to be an increasing awareness of the importance of physical activity amongst younger West Africans, especially men. This is good news and should spur us on to be part of the change we want to see. The bottom line on being active is finding out what works for you and doing it regularly. You know yourself better than anyone else.

Ten Top Tips for a More Active Lifestyle

1. **Discover and do something you enjoy.** Enjoyment is crucial to maintaining the right frequency of activity.
2. **Find an active lifestyle partner.** Having someone hold you accountable and providing support can help your commitment. This could be a friend, family member, work colleague or if you like the gym, your personal trainer.

3. **Take advantage of fitness opportunities at work** if your employer offers them. It may be in the form of use of discounted on-site gym facilities or access to personal trainers.
4. **Decide your fitness goal.** How do you know that you've achieved a goal if you don't even know what it is? Decide if you want to keep healthy, lose weight, tone up, or all three.
5. **Get your dancing shoes on.** Dancing is another fun and inexpensive way to keep fit – especially if you are a guest at a party. You get to tick three boxes all at once: you get your activity in, enjoy yourself in the process and your host/hostess gets the satisfaction of knowing that they hired a great DJ or band.
6. **Want the gym but don't want to commit?** If you are highly motivated and really want to go down the gym route, but membership fees are putting you off, then consider using your local sports or leisure centre on a pay-as-you-use basis.
7. **Bring the gym home.** You can consider hiring gym equipment to use at home with the option of buying at the end of your lease. So if you can't go to the gym but really want to, you can bring the gym to you.
8. **Walk your way to health.** Walking is a good way to start, especially if you have been inactive. It costs nothing and you get a good dose of fresh air whilst doing it. Just remember that a casual stroll won't give you the benefits.
9. **All activity counts – as long as you think FITT.** That includes housework, walking, and gym-based physical exercise.
10. **Be consistent.** The benefits of being active wear off over time if not continued, so keep at it. Remember that no one is perfect, so do cut yourself some slack if things aren't going as you planned – just stick with it.

Activity 3

Research shows that we all tend to overestimate how active we are so to get a more accurate picture, use a pedometer to work out how much you move during the day. Wear your pedometer on your waistband near your hip bone for three or four days and then take an average to get a baseline figure. Your goal is to increase your daily number of steps by 500 steps each week, as a means of moving more and reducing sedentary behaviour. Secondly, you need to sustain your new activity levels. If you are struggling, just remember that any improvement is better than none, and that you are heading in the right direction.

Stress

"If your output is more than your input, your upkeep will be your downfall" – J. John

Are you stressed? Or to put it another way, is life choking the 'life' out of you? Whilst this is not a book on stress management, it is important to understand what stress is and how it can get in the way of your health and ultimately a healthy lifestyle. Stress is an often overlooked but important factor that can have devastating effects on our health. Being stressed is usually associated with work and understandably so, but as you've probably discovered, you can encounter stress anywhere over the course of your day – at the supermarket, at home or at school. A survey carried out by the Relaxation for Living Institute in 2007 showed that one in five of us feels stressed before the day has even started, with the figure doubling by the start of the working day.

We all experience seasons in our lives when everything seems to happen all at once or we have so much to do and so little time in which to do it in. Despite having a multitude of time-saving devices and new technology that promise to make life easier, many of us seem to be left with less time and increasing stress levels. In the UK, seven out of ten visits to the doctor are stress-related, and worryingly, this figure includes both adults and children! The financial impact is just as alarming – in 2005, stress cost the UK economy an estimated £3.7billion and 13 million working days!

It's not all bad news though. Occasional pressure is not a bad thing. In fact, we all thrive on a bit of pressure which motivates us to get things done. The problem arises when we are constantly living in 'pressure cooker' mode which is unsustainable and will ultimately end in stress. Stress is what happens in our minds and bodies when pressure accumulates and our perceived ability to cope is low. In essence, stress is not about what happens to you, but about your perception of your ability to deal with it. Sadly, what goes on in your mind starts to show up in your health. In stressful situations, your body goes into 'fight or flight' mode, releasing a cocktail of hormones to ensure that you are able to respond in an instant. Occasionally this is fine but on a regular basis, you are travelling fast down the highway to high blood pressure, strokes, heart disease, ulcers and even mental health issues.

Another way that uncontrolled stress can have a negative impact on your health is by driving you to indulge in negative behaviours as a means of coping – behaviours such as comfort eating, smoking, drug abuse or some other addiction. It is therefore worth taking measures to keep your stress levels down because you are guaranteed a stressful situation at some point in your life.

Managing Stress

So we know that stress is just one of the unchangeable facts of modern-day life and that we can't avoid it. That said, you can tame this beast. Here are a few strategies that are proven to work:

- **Eat a healthy, balanced diet.** Not surprisingly, as a dietitian I tend to highlight this strategy first because this area of our lives often tends to suffer first when stress strikes. Eating well also helps build your body's resilience to stressful situations by maintaining your immune system.
- **Keep physically fit.** I've already mentioned the fact that regular physical activity helps release endorphins and serotonins - natural 'feel-good' factors which can help improve your mood. It also builds your body's resilience, preparing it to handle stressful situations.
- **Prioritise and learn to say 'No'.** What's important and what's urgent? Realise that saying 'yes' to this in effect means saying 'no' to that.
- **Relax.** Regular time out is important. Switch your phone off, do something you enjoy and relax. Remember that all work and no play makes Jack (or Jill) a dull boy (or girl).
- **Break it down.** Whether it's planning a wedding, dealing with exams or writing a major contract bid, being that bit more organised, planning well and splitting your project into manageable chunks can help you stay on top of things.
- **Be thankful.** No matter how bad things may be, there is always something to be thankful for. Take a few moments each day to identify three things that went well for you. Doing this can help your self-esteem, improve your wellbeing and give you perspective.
- **Get support from friends and family.** This is one strategy that I know as a community we are more than able to deliver on. Our sense of

community spirit is absolutely brilliant because we see each other as an extension of our family, so we rally round each other in times of need.

- **Start the day on a positive note and maintain a positive attitude**. In other words, start as you mean to go on. Are you a 'glass half full' or 'glass half empty' type of person? Do you minimise risk or maximise opportunity? When you are going through a tough time, it's crucial to keep the right perspective. How do you perceive your ability to cope with stressful situations? This will determine your ability to get through stressful times. Remember that it's not what happens to you but how you respond to it that counts.
- **Get professional help.** If stress levels are so high that you are beginning to crumble, then seeking professional help should not be seen as a sign of weakness. It's far less expensive (mentally, emotionally and financially) than a breakdown.

These are only a few strategies and you'll probably have a few others that you find helpful. Applying them will not only help you manage stress but also prevent stress in the first instance. Ask yourself whether you are managing stress or whether it's managing you. If your answer is the latter, you know what to do. Happy stress busting!

Activity 4

Keep a situation and response log, taking some time at the end of each day to reflect on your day. Identify any situations you would classify as stressful (this will vary from person to person). What were your reactions to these situations? Do you notice a trend to how you react? On reflection, how could you respond differently if faced with the same situation again?

Chapter 4

Changing Your Diet And Lifestyle

So far I've explained why we need to change our unhealthy eating and lifestyle habits and how we can achieve change. If you've decided that your diet and lifestyle are not what they should be and that perhaps a few things could do with an overhaul, how do you actually go about changing things? As you probably are aware, it's one thing deciding to change things and quite another to actually 'walk the walk' and make the change.

In considering whether you are ready to take the plunge, you'll need to look at your motivation. What exactly is your reason for wanting to change? Are you intending to change things for genuine reasons, such as your health and wellbeing, or just because it all sounds like a good idea? Feeling guilty about some of the issues raised so far is not a good enough reason to make change. This is a really essential point to consider because it will keep you going, especially when things don't go as planned.

Your readiness to change will depend on: (a) how important you rate the change you want to make, and (b) how confident you are about achieving it. This is because if doing something is really important to you, you'll move heaven and earth to get it done and vice versa. In the same vein, if you are confident in your ability to do something, that confidence will spur you on to do it. The opposite is also true: if a goal is very important to you but you lack the confidence to achieve it, then chances are that you won't pursue it. A quick test to determine the personal importance of changing your diet or lifestyle is to weigh up the benefits and costs of doing so. For example, if you have a family history of high blood pressure, the benefits of making diet and lifestyle changes would include a reduced risk of high blood pressure and stroke. The cost of making these changes would include being more conscious of your eating habits and increasing your physical activity levels. Weighing both the costs and benefits of change will help you decide whether the change you are considering is worth making. If all you can see or think about are the costs of making change, then you might need to wait till you really see the need to do something different. You should also consider the benefits of staying the same i.e. not having to do anything and continuing with life as it is. The cost though could be your health and possibly your life, which, in itself could serve as a wake up call regarding the importance of the matter at hand.

Habits

During your attempt to change areas of your diet and lifestyle, you should expect that things will not all be smooth sailing, especially when the initial enthusiasm wears off - think of all those broken New Year resolutions. Why were they not kept? Here's why: we are creatures of habit and old habits die hard! Think about what you did when you got out of bed first thing this morning. Whatever it was, I can predict that you probably did the same thing yesterday and the day before. Our capacity to do the same things effortlessly over and over again without even realising is amazing. The unfortunate thing about habits is that they can sabotage change by preventing the desire to change. Habits are indeed like a comfortable bed – easy to get into but difficult to get out of. While that's great when the end result is positive, think about what the implications could be when the habit is harmful!

The secret to successful change

Ditching bad habits is about doing things differently and requires a lot of planning and thought. The change you decide to make should also be well thought out so that you clearly know what your goals are and commit to them. This is because change in one area of your life will certainly have an impact on other areas. Therefore, the secret to successful change is preparation. No amount of enthusiasm can make up for this. I mentioned earlier that your confidence level is another key ingredient in successful change. Having the confidence to make change successfully depends on the following: your past experience, getting support from the right people, seeing results, observing or learning from other people's successes and most importantly, practice, practice, practice!

One aim of this book is to help build your confidence by providing you with correct information and useful tools (such as short tasks), to get you to apply what you've learnt. The most important way of becoming confident at doing something is to actually do it. Learning by doing always results in proficiency, in the same way that knowledge only becomes power when you apply it. I hope that by now, this book has made the goal of a healthy diet and lifestyle personal to you and therefore important. The reality is, if you have all the confidence in the world and having a healthy diet and lifestyle is not important to you, you will never achieve it.

Health and habits

Health-wise, habits have a lot to answer for. Prior to making any change to your diet and lifestyle, you will need to take into consideration the effect the change you intend to make will have on different areas of your life. This is because habits rarely exist in isolation - they are often linked to each other. For example, if you are used to eating high calorie snacks whilst watching TV, then you would most likely need to address your TV habits too.

Goal setting

The next thing is to identify how you are going to achieve your goals because intentions only become actions with careful planning. You also need to think about what may get in the way of your goals and what you can do to get around them. Setting **S.M.A.R.T.E.R** goals is an easy way of keeping on top of things and tracking your progress. Your goals need to be:

- **Specific.** What exactly do you want to do or start doing? This will help you monitor your progress.
- **Measurable.** How will you know when you have achieved your goals? This is important because you will need to not only acknowledge your achievement, but reward yourself for getting there.
- **Achievable.** Is this do-able? Setting achievable goals can help you succeed because each successfully accomplished goal gives you the confidence to tackle the next one.
- **Realistic and relevant.** Can you practically achieve this? Better to start with three small goals rather than an impossible one, as unrealistic goals set you up for failure from the very start. Also, you're the expert on you, so choose goals that are relevant to you.

- **Time-specific.** Set yourself deadlines to have accomplished your goals by. This will help motivate you to realising them. Changing habits of a lifetime will take time, so be realistic with your deadlines.
- **Evaluation.** Set a time to regularly review your progress.
- **Reinforcement.** Decide how you will celebrate your success as a means of encouraging yourself to keep on! It doesn't have to be something expensive either. Simply acknowledging your success and patting yourself on the back does much for your confidence.

Keeping at it (even after getting off track)

Forming new habits can take time and requires patience. It means continuing with your new behaviour until it becomes second nature and you begin to do it automatically. If you do something often enough, you become an expert at it and in the process (you've guessed correctly), you form a habit! It is said that it takes between three to six weeks for new behaviour to become second nature to you. Initially, it will take conscious effort on your part to achieve it, but it gets easier with time, requiring less and less of a conscious effort.

At this point I need to talk about relapse. Consider this scenario: you've always wanted to increase your activity levels and had managed to put in one hour on your exercise bike everyday for two weeks. That is up until a few days ago, when you went off track because you had a couple of late nights. You've since given yourself a huge mental 'F' for 'failed' and don't feel like trying again, especially as this is the second time in a month that you've gone off track and you are seriously thinking of giving up altogether. Is this scenario familiar? If it is, then let me say that relapse, or going off track, is a completely normal part of forming new habits or behaviour. (Yes, you read that correctly, there is no typographical error). The key thing about going off track is learning from the experience.

Let me paint another scenario. Think briefly for a moment about a child learning to walk – how long does it take and how many times do they fall? When they do fall, do they sit there and tell themselves, "that's it, this whole walking business is more than I can handle. I'll never get the hang of it, so I'll just keep crawling on all fours as it's so much easier"? No, they keep at it till they've mastered walking such that they do it all the time without thinking about it. Life is all about learning. In the words of John W. Gardner: "there is no learning without some difficulty and fumbling. If you want to keep on learning, you must keep on risking failure - all your life". Being consistent over time will yield results. While the best things in life may be free, putting effort and time into something gives it value and makes success or the end result even sweeter. Remember that you are striving for progress, not perfection – you are only human after all.

Barriers - what could possibly get in the way?

As part of planning to do things differently, you need to consider what may get in the way. From both my personal and professional experience, these are some common barriers that have gotten in the way or may have the potential to do so, particularly from a West African point of view.

Culture

In basic terms, culture can explained as 'what everyone does', and because cultural beliefs and attitudes are part of our identity, we are not likely to want to do things differently. Some West African cultural perceptions, attitudes and beliefs may get in the way when considering dietary or lifestyle changes. A good example would be regarding the association between certain foods and social class. In some communities within Nigeria, mackerel is often viewed as food for people in lower social classes, whilst red meat tends to be associated with those who are better off. I once suggested having mackerel to a UK-based Nigerian gentleman as a means of increasing his omega-3 fat intake. The expression on his face said it all and in the end we settled on salmon, a more expensive oily fish instead. The irony is that mackerel actually contains more omega-3 fats than salmon! Have you ever considered that some of your cultural perceptions or attitudes towards certain foods may mean that you are losing out on great health benefits? Perhaps you need to question your perceptions and attitudes in light of what you've read so far. Are they founded or unfounded?

Tradition

Tradition on the other hand, is 'how it's always been done'. Now, there's nothing wrong with tradition, unless it's getting in the way of our wellbeing. Just because something's always been done in a particular way doesn't make it right or beneficial. And if that's the case, then it's time for change. If traditionally cooked dishes with generous quantities of salt and oil are contributing to the development of obesity and high blood pressure and ultimately strokes, then embracing change is the best thing we can do. It pays to be proactive and prevention is by far better (and less expensive) than cure.

Lack of awareness or ignorance

It is often said that what you don't know cannot harm you. From a health perspective, what you don't know cannot only harm you, it could kill you! Sometimes, traditional dietary and eating habits are not always beneficial to health, and if you are not aware of which ones are helpful and those that are not, it is very likely that you will not do anything about them.

Impractical or unrealistic advice

Have you ever been given advice, which was not only impractical but also virtually impossible? This book intends to spell the end of that. My favourite example is about a client being advised by a healthcare professional to eat boiled yam with its skin on (in the same way you'd eat a jacket potato), in order to increase their fibre intake! Now, while this makes absolute sense since yam skin is high in fibre, it was culturally inappropriate advice, especially as yam peel is sometimes fed to livestock. Needless to say, the patient in question did not heed this piece of advice (you probably wouldn't have either if you were being asked to eat goat feed), and I cannot blame them for doing so. Yam itself is a relatively good source of fibre, providing 3.9g of fibre per 100g, and eating this and other high fibre foods would have been more practical and realistic in addressing this client's low fibre intake.

These are only a few barriers and there may be others. Ask yourself what may be getting in the way of making positive changes to your lifestyle and health. Be as honest with yourself as you can be. Barriers can be overcome, particularly if you anticipate and prepare for them, and remain open to new ways of dealing with them.

Some final thoughts...

Changing a lifelong way of thinking and behaving won't be easy, but it is possible. Changing your diet and lifestyle habits is an investment in your health which will definitely yield you a good return. Be encouraged that no one expects you to change your lifestyle overnight. Many of us put off making positive changes because of the fact that there is some inconvenience involved. If you are struggling with this, then honestly consider what your health may look like if you decided to maintain the status quo. If what springs to mind is not pleasant, then perhaps this could spur you on to make changes so that you can enjoy the health and wellbeing you'd like. As someone put it, two grams of inconvenience now can help avoid two tonnes of inconvenience in the future.

To make effective and lasting change, focus on the benefits of change rather than the initial inconvenience. Remember, if you do the same things, you'll always get the same results! Simple changes are the easiest to maintain in the long-term, so focus on no more than two or three things at a time and concentrate on maintaining them before changing anything else. Finally, remember that making change is an ongoing process that gets easier and easier, especially once you begin to reap the benefits. Never be afraid of trying new ways of doing things – the way it's always been done doesn't always make it beneficial.

Activity 5

Now let's put into practice what we've been talking about. Get a piece of paper and write five diet and lifestyle goals you would like to achieve. They can be as simple as wanting to drink more fluid or walking for at least 10 minutes each day. You now need to ask yourself how important each goal is, as well as how confident you are about actually achieving it. For each goal, rate its importance on a scale of one to ten (1 being not important and 10 being very important). If your importance rating for a particular change is less than 7, then perhaps this is not a goal to work on at the moment, or it is too big a goal and needs to be broken down into a number of smaller goals.

Choose the two or three changes you believe would be easiest to make. These are the ones to focus on because you are more likely to succeed at achieving them, and success, they say, breeds success. Succeeding at these goals will give you the confidence to make the other changes you want to make. Now that you know which of your goals are most important to you, you need to also rate how confident you feel about achieving these goals. Once again, rate these on a scale of one to ten. Confidence-wise, you are more likely to achieve your goal if you have a rating of 5 or more. As I've already mentioned, there are ways to get your confidence levels up so don't worry too much about a score lower than 5. The final step is to make your goals **S.M.A.R.T.E.R** and consider what could get in the way of your plans. Also, have a plan of action for how to overcome any barriers.

Chapter 5

Common Health Problems

West African adults are 13 times more likely to suffer from diabetes and other conditions linked to obesity like hypertension and stroke. The bad news is that the evidence is all around us - we probably all know someone in our family or circle of friends who has one or more of these conditions, or has lost their life as a result of them. The good news is that these conditions can be easily prevented with a few small diet and lifestyle changes.

We are now going to take a look at some of the health conditions which have a high incidence in people of West African origin, to gain a better understanding of them. If you don't suffer from any of these and are striving to eat and live healthily, reading this chapter should strengthen your resolve. If you have already been diagnosed and are living with one or more of these conditions, be encouraged - this chapter intends to help you eat and live better by showing you how to take control of your diet and lifestyle.

Obesity

Obesity has become the fastest growing health problem globally and the greatest public health challenge. Believe it or not, starvation and obesity are both caused by the same thing – poor nutrition, which explains why obesity is classed as malnutrition. Whilst the cause of obesity is not simply attributed to poor nutrition, I hope this view of obesity helps to portray it for what it really is.

Professionally, obesity is of particular interest to me and my experience in obesity management is extensive and varied. I've consulted with individuals, led on community-based weight management programmes, trained other healthcare professionals to treat obesity, and developed and facilitated weight management groups. I have also worked alongside national charities and government agencies, as well as organisations in the commercial slimming and private health insurance industries, to address the problem of obesity. Based on my experience, I think it's time we recognised and tackled the problem of obesity as a community.

Achieving and maintaining a healthy weight is key to dramatically reducing the likelihood of developing obesity-related conditions, which is why I'm addressing obesity first. Obesity increases your chances of developing a range of diseases including diabetes and hypertension, which are already prevalent in people of West African heritage. There is also a very strong link between obesity and cancer, an association recently highlighted in a report by the World Cancer Research Fund.

Measuring overweight and obesity

You can find out whether you are the correct weight or weigh more than you should by working out your body mass index (BMI). The BMI is the international standard for measuring overweight and obesity, but is only a guide. As a calculation, it is simply your body weight (in kilograms) divided by the square of your height (in metres) i.e. BMI = Body weight (Kilograms)/Height^2 (Metres). For adults, a BMI between 20 and 24.9kg/m^2 is categorised as normal; 25-29kg/m^2 is considered overweight; 30kg/m^2 and above is obese. It is important to note that the BMI calculation does not take into account your body composition i.e. how much fat and how much muscle you have. As such, it will not apply to very muscular people such as athletes or bodybuilders because for them, a high BMI will be attributed to muscle (which is denser than fat). Notwithstanding, though the BMI may not be the best indicator of body fat, it is still a good indicator of health risk, and as your BMI increases, your risk of health problems and their severity also increases.

Why are we so heavy?

One of the possible explanations for a high incidence of obesity in the West African community is the perception we often attach to body size – culturally, a more rounded body shape has long been seen as an indicator of an affluent lifestyle and health or wellness. As such, obesity is perceived as a desirable state, indicating strength and affluence in men, and beauty in women. So, while Western cultures attach negativity to being big, in our community being big is often actively celebrated and encouraged, usually unconsciously! So much so, that in some parts of West Africa such as Nigeria and Mauritania, young ladies of marriageable age are customarily 'fattened' over a period of time in preparation for marriage. In Mauritania for instance, the more stretch marks a 'fattened' young lady has, the more desirable she is perceived to be. In essence, within our community, being attractive and being overweight are not mutually exclusive.

It's quite easy to understand why we are so relaxed about something so serious. Weight is not really an issue per se in our community, perhaps because we see it all around us on a daily basis. When you see yourself or loved ones reflected in so many people everyday, it does not bother or surprise you. Rather, you accept it as the norm.

Even if we are conscious of our need to lose weight, we are less inclined to feel pressured to do so compared with our Western counterparts. A larger body image has therefore been accepted as normal - and this seems to resonate within the diverse black communities worldwide. Studies in the United States for instance, show that African-American women are less likely to diet and less fearful of weight gain than white women. Cultural loyalty and a strong ethnic identity are suggested as reasons why this may be the case. In essence, people of African heritage, including West Africans, are culturally comfortable with being a larger size! This cultural acceptance can many times distort the truth of being overweight and its consequences, as well as get in the way of losing excess weight. In fact, amongst West Africans, losing weight is often associated with illness, hardship or poverty.

The high prevalence of overweight and obesity in the West African community suggests a continuous calorie intake exceeding calorie requirements, especially when some of our portion sizes are taken into consideration. Combine this with the less healthy aspects of the Western diet that we've adopted, plus a more sedentary lifestyle and ignorance about the detrimental effects of some traditional eating and cooking habits, and we have a recipe for being overweight without trying too hard.

What makes people gain weight?

While poor eating habits and a sedentary lifestyle are the usual suspects, there is evidence that life events such as getting married, moving in together, having a baby, the menopause, getting older, retirement and stopping smoking are all associated with weight gain. Comfort eating (i.e. using food as a tool to deal with stress and emotional highs and lows), can also make the problem worse. Additionally, having parents who are overweight is a strong risk factor for weight gain.

The cost of obesity

In the UK it is estimated that the National Health Service spends £7.4 billion each year on overweight and obesity, and by 2050 if current trends continue, that estimate is predicted to rise to £46 billion. Obesity is not just expensive in monetary terms, it also has health implications. Obesity is associated with at least forty different health conditions including cancer, heart disease, stroke, diabetes, joint problems, high blood pressure, high cholesterol, and fertility problems (e.g. polycystic ovary syndrome).

The good news is that current evidence shows that modest weight loss of between five and ten percent of your current weight can significantly improve your health, and even add years to your life. Acknowledging the excess weight and not simply dismissing it as being 'big-boned' is a start. Reducing your calorie intake as well as increasing your physical activity, are the two main strategies to get weight loss going. Additionally, you will also need to address the behaviours behind your initial weight gain by getting rid of old, unhelpful habits and forming new, helpful ones. This approach ensures that you re-educate yourself and modify your eating habits and lifestyle - a fool-proof way to sustain your weight loss in the long-term.

Numbers, numbers on the scale

If you are heavier than you should be, those numbers on the scale are simply a reflection of unhelpful and unhealthy behaviours. Let me also add that becoming overweight takes place over a period of time, and so losing weight will also take time. As straightforward as this sounds, it's amazing how many people fall for the latest weight-loss solution. Be wary of 'quick-fix' solutions and fad diets which suggest that you do not have to make long-term changes to your diet and lifestyle to achieve weight loss. The best a quick-fix approach can do is lead to short-term weight loss, with weight regain once you revert to your usual eating habits and food intake. At its worst it can lead to 'yo-yo' dieting which is bad for your long-term general health. To be logical about it, if fad diets were truly as miraculous as claimed, then the problem of obesity would be decreasing and not increasing!

"What about weight loss programmes where meals are replaced with shakes, snack bars and ready-prepared meals?" I hear you say. Well, there shouldn't be a 'one size fits all' approach to weight loss and some of these meal replacement programmes have been successfully used by some people to lose and keep weight off. If you think this approach will work for you, just make sure the programme of your choice also tackles the underlying eating habits that may have caused the weight gain in the first place. Also consider cost – many of these meal replacements can be expensive compared to buying ordinary food.

A very common observation made by people in the process of trying to lose weight is that they initially start to lose weight and then weight loss slows down, even becoming static. This is known as a 'plateau' and is to be expected. In fact, over the time it takes you to reach your target weight, you are likely to experience a number of plateaus. This happens because the minimum amount of energy required for your body to function at rest (your basal metabolic rate or BMR), depends on your body mass or weight. When you lose weight, your body mass decreases as does your BMR, and because your body 'spends' less energy (calories) than it would if you were heavier, the rate of weight loss slows down.

Meet Mrs Coker

Mrs Coker had tried to lose weight over a period of two years without success. Her knees hurt from carrying excess weight and walking short distances left her breathless. Additionally, she was on medication for high blood pressure. She ate regular meals but denied eating large amounts. She did admit that she usually had a packet of reduced-fat crisps after lunch five times a week, while watching her favourite TV show. The specific brand of crisps contained about 100 calories per packet, which was low compared to regular crisps. However, these were calories her body did not need. Consequently, in a week, she was having 500 extra calories, which over the course of a year, added up to more than 25,000 extra calories! Considering that 1kg of body fat is equivalent to 7000 calories, it meant she had gained over 3.5kg over the year from crisps alone. This discovery sparked her decision to really do something about her weight and she willingly cut down to two packets of crisps a week, with the intention of going down to one a week. We agreed on healthier snacks such as fruit. In addition, we addressed the behaviour she associated with eating crisps (i.e. watching TV), by introducing use of her exercise bike while watching TV. This, coupled with other changes, resulted in weight loss of 5kg over 10 weeks, and she remains motivated to reach her target weight of 70kg. Her blood pressure levels have also improved and she can now walk longer distances without breathlessness.

It is usually very easy to become discouraged when experiencing a plateau, especially if the amount of weight you lose serves as your motivation. It can also be even more frustrating when you know you are carefully following your weight loss plan. Since plateaus happen, I think the emphasis when losing weight should be on making and managing lifestyle changes, with the end result or benefit being weight loss – don't focus too much on the amount of weight lost. Also, anticipating and accepting that a plateau is inevitable should serve as extra motivation for you to continue with your plan and reassure you that you are on the right path.

Muscling in on the benefits of physical activity

Increasing your activity levels is a sure way of burning those extra calories; it is also important to include some resistance work as part of your routine, to help build your muscle mass. Muscle tissue plays a really important role in weight control. This is because your body 'spends' more calories to maintain muscle tissue than it does for fat tissue. This is why professional athletes can eat so many calories and not gain weight. As such, increasing your physical activity levels can help overcome plateaus. Light to moderate resistance work won't turn you into a bodybuilder and you don't necessarily have to use weights, as your body can provide all the resistance required. All you have to do is work against this resistance.

Weight maintenance, the most important part of losing weight, can also prove to be the most challenging. Maintaining your new weight is a long-term indicator of your success and should be an ongoing part of your new lifestyle.

Ten Top Tips for Successful Weight Loss

Here are some tips to not only aid weight loss, but also help to keep it off:

1. **Are you really ready to lose weight?** Studies show that for successful weight loss to happen you need to be ready mentally, as well as committed to losing weight; otherwise you set yourself up for failure right from the start.

2. **Ditch the diet and sign up for the long haul.** Accept that weight loss takes time; there are no long-lasting quick fixes. Fad diets don't work because they tend to be rigid and inflexible. Instead, make small, lasting changes which you can realistically manage.
3. **Set a realistic target weight**. Split your weight loss target into smaller, realistic and achievable targets. Aim for sensible weight loss of half to 1 kg (1 to 2lbs) per week.
4. **Watch portion sizes.** Forget calorie counting which can be complex. If you are struggling with large portion sizes, use a smaller plate than you would normally use. Visually divide your plate into four and fill it as follows: two quarters vegetables, a quarter meat, fish or alternative protein, and a quarter starchy foods. Put food on your plate in that order and in those proportions. See Chapter 2 for how this applies to meals with West African soups and stews.
5. **Keep a food diary.** This can help you learn more about yourself, your habits and relationship with food, as well as any associated thoughts and feelings. You can use this as a tool to work out what dietary changes you need to make.
6. **Have breakfast.** Research shows that people who eat breakfast tend to be more successful at losing weight than those who do not. This is because if you skip breakfast, you are more likely to assuage your hunger with high-calorie convenience foods or over-compensate with the other meals you have during the rest of the day. Aim to eat within 2 hours of waking up.
7. **Hit a plateau?** If your weight loss has become static, the most important thing you can do is to continue with your healthy eating plan and step up your

activity levels. Stepping up your activity levels can be very useful because it increases your muscle mass and uses up calories.

8. **Get moving!** Try using a pedometer to keep track of the number of steps you take daily and aim to move more each day. Exercise or activity can also help you eat less by taking your mind off food. Chemical substances called endorphins are released during physical activity and help improve your mood.
9. **Carbs are not the enemy, too many calories are**. Starchy foods (a.k.a. carbohydrates or carbs) are not fattening –unless you drown them in fat or eat large quantities of them. In the right amounts they help satisfy your appetite without too many calories (for comparison, carbohydrates contain 4 calories per gram while fats contain 9 calories per gram). Furthermore, not eating an adequate amount of carbs makes it difficult for you to be physically active, as your muscles prefer carbs for their fuel.
10. **Celebrate success, no matter how small.** Each kilogram or pound in weight that you lose takes you a step closer to your target weight, so it's worth shouting about it. Reward your achievements - it may be a movie, a mini-chocolate bar or a pampering session. Use non-food rewards if food rewards are simply temptation waiting to happen.

Diabetes

Diabetes is a lifelong condition in which the body does not produce or properly use insulin, a hormone needed to control the conversion of food into energy. When starchy or sugary foods are eaten and digested, they are broken down into glucose, a natural sugar which is used to meet the body's energy requirements. Insulin helps to maintain levels of glucose in the blood, ensuring they are not too high or too low, but remain within a normal range of 4-7 milimoles of glucose per litre of blood. Insulin acts like a key, allowing glucose into the body's cells where it is used as energy for normal cell activity. The body not producing enough insulin, or not using it properly, is equivalent to not having keys, or having keys that do not work. The result of this is an accumulation of glucose in the blood.

At present there is no cure for diabetes but it can be managed by maintaining a healthy lifestyle, (including diet and exercise) and taking appropriate medication. There are 3 main types of diabetes:

- **Type 1 Diabetes**, which happens when the pancreas does not make any insulin at all. It is more common in adolescents and young adults, accounting for about 5-15% of all diabetes cases. Treatment involves dietary education as well as insulin replacement via injections, pumps or inhalers.
- **Type 2 Diabetes**, which is the most prevalent type of diabetes, accounts for more than 85-95% of all diabetes cases and is more common in adults and the elderly. It develops when the pancreas does not make enough insulin, or if there is insulin resistance - a situation where there is sufficient insulin but it is not recognised. Treatment involves dietary education, and in most cases, tablets and/or insulin.
- **Gestational Diabetes** occurs in pregnancy when the body cannot meet the increased demand for insulin caused by the growing baby and hormones your body makes. When this happens, blood glucose levels rise above normal. Treatment of gestational diabetes is usually by dietary education and if that fails, insulin. Whilst this type of diabetes disappears after delivery, there is an increased risk of developing Type 2 diabetes later in life.

What causes Type 2 Diabetes?

Since Type 2 diabetes is a growing problem in the West African community, we need to understand what increases our risk of developing this condition so we can actively and knowledgeably reduce our risk. Contrary to popular belief, diabetes is not caused by consuming too much sugar. Rather, there are a number of factors that can play a role in increasing the risk of developing diabetes. These include:

- **Overweight or obesity:** The majority (about 4 out of 5) of all people with Type 2 diabetes are obese. With excess weight, body cells can become insulin resistant or cannot effectively use the insulin your body makes. Carrying excess weight around your waist further increases your risk of developing diabetes, so it is important to be aware of your waist circumference or measurement. A waist measurement of less than 94cm (37 inches) for black men and less than 80cm (31.5 inches) for black women is healthy.
- **Family history:** A family history of diabetes increases your risk of developing the condition. For example, the risk of developing diabetes if one parent has Type 2 diabetes is 14%; this becomes 75% if both parents have Type 2 diabetes.
- **Age:** On average, most Type 2 diabetes patients are over 40 years old at diagnosis but this can be slightly earlier in people of West African origin. Diagnosis of diabetes at an earlier age is higher in the obese, those with a family history of diabetes, and those leading sedentary lifestyles.
- **Race:** In the UK, West Africans are 13 times more likely to develop this type of diabetes than the UK national average. People of other ethnic backgrounds also have a high risk.

- **A history of gestational diabetes** in a woman increases her likelihood of developing permanent diabetes later in life.

The best way to reduce your risk of diabetes is to put into practice the diet and lifestyle principles we've discussed so far in previous chapters. If the risk factors above have already caught up with you and you have diabetes, it may come as a pleasant surprise that the dietary advice for people with diabetes is no different from the advice for people without diabetes. Simply put, it's healthy eating all the way, with a few straightforward modifications which I'll explain in more detail a little later.

Symptoms

It is estimated that over 2 million people in the UK have diabetes, whilst a further 750,000 are yet to be diagnosed. Even more alarming is the fact that the majority of these will be Type 2 diabetes which can have serious long-term complications such as blindness, limb amputations, kidney failure and an increased risk of strokes and heart attacks. Considering that as a community we have an increased risk of developing Type 2 diabetes, we need to improve our awareness of symptoms that may point towards the presence of undiagnosed (or poorly controlled diabetes) including:

- Passing large amounts of urine frequently
- Excessive thirst accompanied with a dry mouth
- Extreme tiredness and lack of energy
- Weight loss
- Blurred vision
- Frequent infections e.g. thrush, cystitis, boils

- Burning or a 'pins and needles' sensation in legs.
- Ketones in the urine (only in Type 1 diabetes) – indicates that blood glucose levels are dangerously high, needing urgent treatment. If left untreated, this can result in diabetic coma. One tell-tale sign of this symptom is breath smelling of fruit or nail polish remover.

Diagnosis

Early diagnosis makes such a difference because it ensures effective treatment. Statistics in the UK show that along with people of South Asian and Caribbean origin, diabetes in people of West African origin is less likely to be detected, and when diagnosed, less likely to be adequately treated. Diabetes is diagnosed by one or more of three laboratory blood tests: a random blood glucose test, a fasting blood glucose test and an oral glucose tolerance test. The different test results should be explained to you when the diagnosis is made. Be aware that diabetes is an 'all or nothing' condition like pregnancy - you either have it or don't. Furthermore, there is no such thing as having a 'touch of diabetes', as some clients have been told upon diagnosis. Furthermore, there is nothing 'mild' about Type 2 diabetes (compared to Type 1) either. In fact, it is a very serious condition and should be considered as such.

Treatment

Though diabetes is a serious condition, it can be treated and controlled. Coming to terms with the diagnosis and taking responsibility for or ownership of your diabetes, are the first steps towards managing it successfully. Secondly, treatment or management should be a joint effort between yourself and your designated healthcare professional(s).

Sometimes, diabetes can be controlled by diet alone, but in many cases medication (tablets or insulin) is prescribed. Always remember to take your medication if you are on any at all and follow the instructions given. They play an important role in controlling your blood sugar levels and therefore reduce your risk of long-term complications. An active lifestyle with frequent exercise is also known to make your body use insulin better and help in controlling blood sugar levels.

Hypoglycaemia

Hypoglycaemia, or a 'hypo', is the medical term for low blood sugar levels and tends to be experienced by people treated with insulin or particular diabetic tablets. Common causes of hypoglycaemia are:

- Taking too much insulin or diabetes medication
- Drinking alcohol on an empty stomach
- Missing or delaying a meal or snack
- Being more physically active than usual

So how do you know you are having a hypo? Common warning signs include feeling faint or light-headed, sweating, shaking, being irritable, hunger and confusion. Bear in mind that this will vary from person to person. Treating a hypo involves eating or drinking something sugary (e.g. three to six glucose tablets, 50-100ml of lucozade or 200ml of fruit juice), to quickly raise blood sugar levels. This should be followed by eating something more substantial such as a banana, a slice of toast or a glass of milk, to maintain the improved blood glucose level.

Diet and diabetes

In addition to any medication you may be prescribed (i.e. tablets or insulin), looking after your diet remains the cornerstone of managing your diabetes. A good diet can prevent the damage that can occur as a result of persistently high or uncontrolled blood glucose levels. There is no such thing as a 'diabetic diet' and there is no need to avoid sugar completely. A sugar-free diet is virtually impossible to achieve as some sugars occur naturally in most foods; you simply need to monitor your sugar intake and be aware of foods and drinks which are high in natural and added sugars.

West African foods that may help with diabetes

Many popularly eaten traditional West African foods have health benefits when eaten as part of a healthy balanced diet. Though this potential has remained untapped, emerging research is beginning to showcase their great but not widely known health benefits. Here are some traditional West African foods that may help with diabetes:

- **Leafy vegetables and soup thickeners**: A recent Nigerian study involving newly diagnosed Type 2 diabetes patients on tablets, found that a diet high in fibre provided by leafy vegetables and soup thickeners (tallow tree seeds and horse eye beans), resulted in a reduction of both blood glucose and blood cholesterol levels. Whilst it was a small study, these findings have been corroborated by ongoing research at King's College, University of London. This research at King's College indicates that soluble fibre in tallow tree seeds shows considerable promise in the treatment of diabetes and hyperlipidaemia, as it lowers both blood glucose and blood cholesterol levels. The findings of both these studies are not surprising considering that the lowering effects of both soluble and insoluble fibre on blood glucose and blood cholesterol levels are already well known.

- **Okra**: The high soluble fibre content of okra could help stabilise blood sugar levels in diabetes, because it may reduce the rate at which sugars are absorbed from the intestine.
- **Fonio and millet porridges**: Research has shown that, when compared to other cereals, both fonio and millet have lower glycaemic indices. Consequently, they could help regulate blood sugar levels as the rate at which their natural sugars are released into the blood stream is slower than that of some other cereals.

Fasting and Diabetes

Fasting is often an integral part of the religions and faiths that many West Africans embrace. For example, fasting is a discipline of both Christianity and Islam, two of the main faiths common in our community. Whilst it is actually possible for the majority of people with Type 2 diabetes to fast safely, this should only be done with the agreement and backing of your healthcare team. This is because some types of diabetes medication (specifically sulphonylureas and insulin), can make your blood sugar levels become dangerously low. You will usually be assessed to ensure that you are in good condition to fast - any long-term complications, such as damage to the eyes, kidneys or the nerves in your hands and feet, will compromise your ability to fast.

If your diabetes is well controlled, your healthcare team may be able to change the time and dose of your medication (including insulin), enabling you to fast for a certain period of time. You will also be advised to follow a healthy eating plan. A light meal before dawn is advised to prevent low blood sugar levels during the day, and you need to drink a good amount of fluid to prevent dehydration.

Ten Top Tips for Eating Well with Diabetes

1. **Aim to eat 3 regular meals every day**. This will help to control your appetite and blood glucose levels.
2. **Base each meal on starchy carbohydrate foods**. Aim to eat a variety of starchy foods, especially ones that are absorbed more slowly i.e. have a lower GI (glycaemic index) e.g. pasta, basmati rice, unripe plantain, sweet potatoes and yam. See Chapter 2 for more information on starchy foods.
3. **Eat more fruit and vegetables**. Aim for at least 3 portions of fruit and 2 portions of vegetables daily. Fruit is naturally sweet so spread your fruit portions out over the day and have only one portion of fruit at a time. This will prevent high blood sugar levels. Also, limit fruit juice to one small glass (150ml or 5 fluid ounces) a day with a meal.
4. **Cut down your intake of fat especially saturated fat** (e.g. fatty meats, butter and palm oil). Choose unsaturated fats, preferably monounsaturated fats like olive or rapeseed oil. Also, choose lower fat dairy products and use fat-free cooking methods.
5. **Limit your intake of sugary foods and drinks.** Try using an artificial sweetener instead and have sugar-free, diet or no-added sugar squashes instead of ordinary versions. Limit sugary drinks (such as malt drinks) to about half a bottle (about 165ml) occasionally. Also, drink this with a meal to prevent your blood glucose levels rising too quickly.
6. **Aim for at least 2 portions of oily fish a week.** These contain omega-3 fats which help look after your heart. Salmon, sardines, pilchards and mackerel are good sources, as are *bonga fish*, giant snails and tropical periwinkles.
7. **Eat more beans and pulses.** These contain soluble fibre which will help control your blood glucose levels as well as cholesterol levels.

8. **Reduce salt intake to 6g or less a day.** This includes salt added to foods as well as salt that is naturally present in foods. 6g is equivalent to just over one teaspoonful.
9. **Drink alcohol in moderation** and remember that drinking on an empty stomach can cause low blood sugar levels (hypoglycaemia).
10. **Diabetic foods or drinks are not beneficial.** They are expensive and if consumed in excess, can have a laxative effect, as well as lead to weight gain.

High blood pressure: The silent killer

The British Heart Foundation estimates that 5.3 million people in the UK do not know they have high blood pressure. A lifelong disease, high blood pressure is also known as the 'silent killer' because, although no signs indicate its presence, it can have devastating effects if not diagnosed, treated and controlled. For example, untreated high blood pressure can result in other serious health conditions such as stroke, heart disease, kidney disease and in men, erectile dysfunction. People with high blood pressure are three times more likely to develop heart disease and stroke, and twice as likely to die from these diseases compared to those with normal blood pressure levels. High blood pressure is said to be present when a person's blood pressure reading measures more than 140/80mmHg[4].

---

[4] MmHg - a measure of pressure

What causes high blood pressure?

Research suggests that people of African heritage have a higher risk of developing high blood pressure. This is thought to be due to an increased sensitivity to the hypertensive effect of salt. Africans are therefore at an increased risk of developing stroke, heart and kidney disease. In addition to being genetically predisposed to developing high blood pressure, some of our dietary habits worsen our risk, the main one being our love of salt - which many of us are addicted to. As West Africans, we say food tastes bland without added salt and so, we liberally sprinkle it into our cooking and, in some cases, add more at the table. Many of us are unaware of the different sources of salt in our diet. We freely use salt-based seasonings (like stock cubes, bouillon cubes and all-purpose seasoning) in our cooking. As such, heavily seasoned foods such as stews, meats and poultry tend to be major sources of salt. Smoked and salted fish and meats also contribute.

Research by the Food Standards Agency (FSA) in the UK shows that we are not alone in our love for salt. Current figures reveal that the average amount of salt consumed by men and women is 11g and 8.1g respectively. These figures are much higher than the UK government's recommendation of 6g - just over one teaspoon per day for adults. This recommended figure takes into consideration salt added to food during its preparation, salt found in processed foods (where it is often used as a preservative), as well as salt naturally present in foods in the form of sodium.

In addition to a high salt intake and genetics, here are some other factors that also increase your risk of developing high blood pressure:

- **Overweight.** The more you weigh, the harder your heart has to work to pump blood through excess body tissues, creating higher blood pressure in the process.

- **Age.** The process of ageing increases blood pressure.
- **Stress** elevates blood pressure levels, and chronic or long-term stress compounds this effect.
- **A sedentary lifestyle** with low levels of physical activity.

Symptoms and Diagnosis

You can't 'feel' high blood pressure so most people with high blood pressure don't have any symptoms, or know they have an abnormally high blood pressure level. Consequently, it's extremely important to have regular blood pressure checks. If you have very high blood pressure, or a rapid rise in blood pressure, you may have headaches, problems with your vision, fits, or black-outs.

Ten Top Tips to Manage and Prevent High Blood Pressure

1. **Know your numbers**. Get your blood pressure checked regularly, men especially. Some recent research by Ipsos-MORI in the UK revealed that West African men perceived themselves as having a lower risk of high blood pressure and as a result, were among the least likely to get their blood pressure checked. They also had less awareness of the impact of high blood pressure on their health.
2. **Lose weight.** If you are overweight, losing between 5-10% of what you currently weigh will make a dramatic difference to your blood pressure levels. (See earlier section on obesity for how to determine if you are overweight, as well as for advice on managing your weight).
3. **Keep stress under control**. Stress or pressure is an everyday part of life and can be beneficial if harnessed and managed well. However, experienc-

ing stress on a never-ending basis, or beyond your ability to cope can be harmful to your health in more ways than can be imagined.

4. **Reduce your salt intake.** Studies show that reducing salt in the diet can lower blood pressure within four weeks and may help people on anti-hypertensive drugs to stop medication. The main culprits are foods that are high in salt (or sodium), such as monosodium glutamate-based seasonings (e.g. Maggi, Ajinomoto), salted nuts, processed foods (e.g. tinned meat such as corned beef), crisps, biscuits and packet soups. Sea salt, garlic salt and indigenous rock salt (*kaun* or *kawe*), are almost identical to salt, and should be used in small quantities or not at all. Also, if salt-based seasonings such as all-purpose seasoning are used in cooking, they should be used sparingly. Alternatively, use reduced-salt stock cubes or traditional flavour enhancers like *ogiri* (fermented egusi or castor oil seeds) and *dawadawa* (fermented locust beans).
5. **Eat more fruit and vegetables.** These are naturally high in potassium, known to help lower blood pressure levels. Additionally, many green leafy West African vegetables are rich calcium, which has also been proven to help lower blood pressure. Aim for at least 5 portions daily. See Chapter 2 for portion sizes.
6. **Increase your physical activity levels.** Being physically active can help you maintain a healthy weight and therefore reduce blood pressure levels. It is also a great way to get rid of stress, as your body releases 'feel good factors' or endorphins in response to exercise.
7. **Watch your alcohol intake.** Regularly drinking large amounts of alcohol can raise blood pressure levels. Drink sensibly within the recommended

guidelines of no more than three units per day for men and no more than two units per day for women. See Chapter 7 for more information on this.

8. **Comply with medication if it has been prescribed for you**. Remember that medication will only work if it is taken as prescribed.
9. **Watch your waist.** This is another way of being aware of your weight. A waist measurement of less than 94cm (37 inches) for men and 80cm (31.5 inches) for women is associated with reduced risk of developing high blood pressure.
10. **Start prevention early.** Seeing that as a community, we are at increased risk of developing high blood pressure, let's give the next generation a heads up by starting them on the right path. Explain the negative impact that too much salt can have on health. Take the salt shaker off the table and discourage automatically adding salt to food without tasting.

Prostate Cancer

Prostate cancer is now the most common form of cancer in men in the UK, with more and more men being diagnosed each year. Current figures indicate that almost 32,000 men are diagnosed with prostate cancer each year. The prostate is a walnut-sized gland that plays a role in semen production. Abnormal changes in a few cells in the prostate can result in uncontrolled growth and therefore in its enlargement.

Studies show that men of African descent are at an increased risk of developing prostrate cancer, accounting for the high incidence of this type of cancer in West African men. The Prostate Cancer in Ethnic Subgroups (PROCESS) study showed that death rates from prostate cancer are raised in Caribbean and West African men. It also showed that black men in the United Kingdom have a substantially greater risk of developing prostate cancer compared with white men. The similar rates in black Caribbean and black African men suggest a common genetic cause, although migration may be associated with an increased risk attributable to a gene-environment interaction. Two other factors that can increase your risk are:

- **Age.** This is the strongest risk factor for developing prostate cancer because the prostate gland enlarges with age. There is very low risk in men under the age of 50, increasing thereafter.
- **Family history.** Having a close male relative (father, brother, son) diagnosed with prostate cancer increases your risk, especially if they were diagnosed before the age of 60.

Symptoms and diagnosis

Experiencing any of these should prompt you to see your doctor:

- Increased frequency of urinating, particularly at night.
- Difficulty urinating.
- Stopping and starting while urinating.
- A not-completely-emptied feeling after urinating.
- Having to rush to the toilet to urinate.
- Dribbling urine.

Rather than wait for any of these symptoms to develop, a safer alternative is to have a yearly screening examination by your doctor. A digital rectum examination (DRE) can help determine whether the prostate is enlarged or not, before any of the obvious symptoms come to light. In addition, a prostatic specific antigen (PSA) blood test can also detect prostate cancer. Both these tests can be requested at your doctor's practice and should be requested if you experience any of the above symptoms.

Men are known to have reduced contact with health services and are less likely to seek help even when it's needed. Did you know that almost half of all prostate cancers are detected too late? This isn't because the cancer spreads too fast but because men are slower in making an appointment to see their doctor. If you are over forty and have never attended a screening appointment, don't put it off another day – it could save your life.

Ten Top Tips to Prevent and Manage Prostate Cancer

Some of the steps you can take to reduce your risk of prostate cancer are:

1. **Get yourself screened** or take advantage if screening is offered. Whilst it may be embarrassing and uncomfortable, screening is an effective way of detecting any changes to the prostate gland, thereby stopping the devastating effects of cancer in its tracks.
2. **Monitor yourself** and be aware of any changes in urinating habits. You are the expert on you.
3. **Find out about your family history.**
4. **Don't ignore symptoms and do not delay if you do notice changes.** Many men ignore symptoms or delay contact with their doctor when sick or in pain. There is nothing macho about avoiding a visit to your doctor.
5. **Quit smoking.** Research shows that smokers are three times more likely to be diagnosed with prostate cancer than non-smokers.
6. **Reduce your fat intake, especially saturated fat, and go easy on the meat.** A high fat intake is associated with an increased risk of pros-

tate cancer so reduce your intake of animal products like red meat and full-fat dairy products, as well as palm and coconut oils. Instead choose fish (especially oily fish) more often, eat leaner cuts of red meat when you do, and choose lower-fat dairy products. Studies also associate an increased risk of prostate cancer with a high consumption of red meat, especially processed or charcoal-grilled meats.

7. **Increase your lycopene intake**. Lycopene, the red pigment responsible for the colour of watermelon and tomatoes, is a carotenoid which has been shown to dramatically reduce the risk of prostate cancer. Cooking increases the availability of lycopene, so tomato-based stews and sauces are a good way of having a good lycopene intake. Other sources include red guava and pink grapefruit.
8. **Have an adequate selenium intake.** Low levels of selenium are associated with an increased risk of prostate cancer. Good selenium sources include wholemeal bread and poultry, as well as shellfish such as tropical oysters, prawns and tropical periwinkles.
9. **Maintain a healthy weight.** Excess weight is a risk factor for many cancers, including prostate cancer.
10. **Keep active.** Being active will help to regulate your weight.

Stroke

According to figures from the UK Health Protection Agency, the rate of premature death from stroke for non-UK born West Africans living in the UK is nearly three times higher for men, and 81% higher for women, compared to the rest of the population. These figures are consistent with the high incidence of stroke among

West Africans in the UK. They also reflect our higher than average blood pressure levels, as well as the high prevalence of stroke in many West African countries.

High blood pressure is the most important risk factor for stroke – it promotes the thickening of artery walls by the build-up of fatty material such as cholesterol. Similarly, consistently high blood glucose levels in uncontrolled diabetes can narrow the arteries. In either case, when blood flow is restricted, blood pressure increases, making it easier for the artery to get clogged or burst. A stroke occurs when an artery in the brain gets clogged or bursts. The oxygen supply to the affected part of the brain is cut off, resulting in the death of brain cells in that area. Since the brain is the control tower of the body, if some cells die, then the body parts that these particular cells control stop functioning.

Symptoms

- Speech problems
- Visual problems
- Facial weakness
- Arm or leg weakness or paralysis on one side of the body

In the event that you suspect that someone has had a stroke, a simple and effective way to assess this is by remembering the first 3 letters of 'stroke' i.e. **STR**:

S – Ask the person to smile

T – Ask them to talk i.e. to repeat a simple sentence e.g. "It's raining today".

R – Ask them to raise both arms.

If they fail any one of these three tests, you must call the emergency services immediately so that the person can be taken to hospital quickly for early treatment. Remember that time is of the essence. If signs of stroke only last a few minutes or a few hours, then a Transient Ischemic Attack (TIA) or mini-stroke may have occurred. A TIA is a warning sign that must never be ignored. Seek urgent medical attention for assessment and treatment.

Ten Top Tips for Preventing Stroke

The best way to prevent a stroke is to reduce the risk factors associated with it. Here are some top tips to do this:

1. **Get your blood pressure checked**. What you do not know can actually (and literally) kill you.
2. **Stop smoking.** Smoking causes arteries to become hardened and more easily blocked. It also makes the blood stickier, increasing the risk of blood clot formation in the arteries. Stopping smoking can actually reduce your risk of having a stroke by 50%.
3. **Maintain a healthy weight.** Being overweight increases your risk of diabetes, high blood pressure and heart disease, all of which increase your risk of stroke.
4. **Eat more fruit and vegetables.** According to the World Health Organisation, low fruit and vegetable intake is responsible for 11% of strokes worldwide. Fruit and vegetables are rich in antioxidants which are thought to protect against stroke.
5. **Avoid a high salt intake.** It has been estimated that a reduction in current dietary salt intake to the recommended 6g per day would result in a 13% reduction in stroke.
6. **Consume alcohol in safe quantities.** Regularly drinking large amounts of alcohol can raise blood pressure levels and drinking large amounts at one time (binge drinking) can raise blood pressure to dangerously high levels.

7. **Eat more fish, especially oily fish.** Oily fish is a good source of omega-3 fatty acids which have been proven to naturally thin the blood (preventing blood clots), and lower HDL (bad) cholesterol levels, both of which are implicated in the development of stroke. Other sources of omega-3 fatty acids include giant snails and tropical periwinkles.
8. **Increase your activity levels.** People who are less active are more predisposed to suffering from a stroke than people who do regular moderate exercise.
9. **Watch your fat intake, especially saturated fat.** Saturated fat increases HDL (bad) cholesterol levels which can result in artery damage, and too much fat overall can contribute to weight gain. To reduce your saturated fat intake, swap fatty red meat for leaner cuts, take skin off poultry and use low-fat dairy products.
10. **Speak with your doctor about the combined contraceptive pill and hormone replacement therapy (HRT).** These hormone treatments may increase the risk of high blood pressure and can also make the blood stickier and more likely to clot. Speaking with your doctor will ensure that you make an informed decision.

Chapter 6

Adapting Recipes

In keeping with our strong oral tradition, recipes for popular West African dishes have been handed down verbally over the years. As such, West African cooking is instinctive in nature; our dishes are cooked from experience, guided by our senses of smell and taste. We intuitively recognise what works and what doesn't, and because we know that the combination of certain ingredients can make (or break) a dish, we are more inclined to stick with tradition. But is tradition stealthily compromising our health?

As we've seen already in Chapter 2, many of our foods are bursting with nutrients and health-promoting goodness, so you'll be pleased to know that you don't have to give up your favourite dishes in order to improve your health. They are after all, an integral part of our heritage and identity – there aren't many West Africans who would consider not serving traditional dishes such as *jollof rice*, *oleleh* or *chicken yassa* at their function. We can however take a healthier approach in preparing and serving these dishes and in the process, improve on the culinary traditions that we, (like our ancestors), will pass on to our children one day.

Many of our dishes are composite dishes i.e. dishes containing a mixture of foods from the different food groups. Since our health can be compromised by the way we prepare these dishes because we don't usually cook from written recipes, I have taken the approach of providing suggestions for healthier West African cooking. The aim is to enable you to prepare more healthful dishes and avoid the pitfalls associated with some traditional cooking methods. This in turn will ensure that you begin to take charge of your health right from your kitchen.

Your taste buds may initially protest and some of these suggestions may seem to go against conventional West African cooking practices, but try them at least and see. What's there to lose? You might draw some inspiration and be pleasantly surprised in the process. Besides, your health will thank you for it. For readers who prefer a more precise and measured approach, I've also included a few healthy recipes of my own for you to try, as a means of inspiring you towards healthier cooking. These healthier versions of some popular West African dishes have been nutritionally analysed to provide vital information regarding their calorie and nutritional content.

Suggestions for healthier West African cooking

Here are some ideas on how to prepare and serve our dishes, making them less likely to contribute to ill health:

- Cook with less oil by making a conscious effort to measure how much you use rather than pouring straight from the bottle. Alternatively, use a spray oil.
- Use less palm oil and more tomato purée and puréed red sweet peppers instead, for an appetising colour and less saturated fat.
- Avoid adding butter or margarine to boiled rice prior to serving.
- For dishes requiring coconut milk, use 'reduced-fat' or 'light' versions.
- Prior to use, soak dried, smoked fish in hot water to get rid of sand and grit, as well as some of the salt content. This kind of fish is usually salted prior to smoking to preserve it.

- Likewise, soak salt fish and salt meats (such as beef and pork) overnight prior to use, to remove salt. High salt intakes can raise blood pressure levels and increase the risk of stomach cancer.
- Serve pulses and legumes as part of a dish to help reduce meat portions. Legumes, nuts and seeds are good sources of protein and can therefore be used as alternatives for meat, which can be high in saturated fat. Additionally, they are packed with polyphenols, lignans and fibre which are all protective against cancer.
- Avoid frying meat and fish, either to eat on its own or for use in soups and stews. Rather, dry roast them in the oven or under the grill, making sure to use the grid. This allows the fat to drip off, ensuring that it is not reabsorbed. Alternatively, lightly crisp lean, boiled meat in the microwave for quick and easy crispiness without the added fat (and calories).
- Lightly cooking vegetables preserves their nutritional value. When cooking dishes requiring vegetables, add vegetables right at the end of cooking so that they are cooked by the residual heat.
- Wash vegetables before cutting, bruising or shredding, to preserve their nutrient content. Remember to always cook for minimum time and in as little water as possible, because vitamin C is sensitive to heat and is water-soluble.
- Incorporating homemade stocks into dishes is a good way of boosting the iron content of a dish as some iron from the meat is left in the stock. Use a small amount (1 or 2 tablespoons) of lemon juice or vinegar when pre-cooking large quantities of meat on the bone, to help extract calcium and other minerals from the bone. Drain the stock, refrigerate it and skim fat off before from it using it for cooking.

- Do not 'bleach' palm oil by heating it to high temperatures – you lose the beta-carotene which is responsible for its orange colour and which the body converts into vitamin A, a powerful antioxidant.
- If frying cannot be avoided, use a good quality vegetable oil, such as corn, soya, groundnut (peanut), sunflower, or rapeseed oils. Frequently change the oil in your fryer to reduce the risk of trans fatty acid formation, which happens when cooking oils are heated to high temperatures. In addition, food should be cut into larger, thicker pieces as this reduces surface area and consequently reduces the amount of oil absorbed. Remember to limit how much and how often fried food is eaten.
- Add some vinegar or lemon juice to marinades for meat when grilling or barbequing to prevent the formation of heterocyclic amines, potential cancer causing substances which are formed when meat is cooked at very high temperatures.
- Consider baking chin-chin instead of frying.
- Use traditional fermented condiments such as *dawadawa* and *ogiri* to enhance the flavours of dishes. Take into account that some versions of *ogiri* may contain salt as a preservative.
- Use traditional herbs and spices instead of large quantities of salt to liven up dishes. Many traditional West African herbs and spices are aromatic in nature and bursting with phenols which have antioxidant properties. Country onion for example, a popular Cameroonian spice, has an amazing flavour and aroma which is sure to make any dish sing. Milled *crayfish* is also a great flavour enhancer.
- Swap your usual stock cubes for reduced-salt versions and follow instructions found on packaging of commercial seasonings. For example, one

popular brand of all-purpose seasoning recommends the use of 1 teaspoon of seasoning per half kilo of meat.

- Most sauces used at the table are also very high in salt, e.g. chilli sauces, tomato ketchup and soy sauce. Therefore, look for reduced salt versions or use them sparingly. Reduced sodium salts, such as Lo-Salt, Solo and So-Low, as well as salt substitutes like Ruthmol, are not recommended.
- Refrain from adding salt to plantain or yam before frying them.
- Marinate meat and fish in food bags or Ziploc bags with salt-free seasoning and leave in the freezer. They'll be full of flavour when you're ready to cook.
- Trim off visible fat from meat or skin from poultry before cooking - this stops the fat from soaking into the meat during cooking.
- Skim off excess oil from traditionally oily dishes such as *palm butter*, *torbogee* and groundnut soups before serving.
- As a means of keeping the calories down, use cooking methods which do not require fat or oil such as grilling, boiling, microwaving and steaming. To illustrate how much of a difference this can make, take a look at this table:

Nutrition Information per 100g	**Snapper (Fish)**		**Plantain**		**Chicken**	
	Fried	**Steamed**	**Fried**	**Boiled**	**Fried**	**Roast**
Calories	276	149	267	112	242	148
Fat	17	9	9	0	13	5

- Using a pressure cooker to cook beans shortens cooking time and preserves their nutritional quality. Studies have shown that while adding indigenous rock salt (*kaun, kangwa*) speeds up cooking time, it also causes high losses of vitamins B_1 (thiamin) and B_2 (riboflavin), even when small quantities are used. Using indigenous rock salt also reduces the levels of certain amino acids in beans.

- Boiling (but not overcooking), steaming and cooking in the microwave, are great ways to preserve the nutritional content of vegetables.
- Use a non-stick pan to 'dry-fry' eggs.
- Using a mix of dried and fresh leafy green vegetables in cooking will help you get their maximum benefit since dried varieties have a higher phytochemical content while fresh vegetables contain more vitamins.
- To improve intake of leafy vegetable portions, try preparing your vegetable soup as usual, but leave out the vegetables. Steam your vegetables in the microwave till just cooked and add the equivalent of 6 heaped tablespoons or 1½ cooking spoons of the vegetables to each adult portion of soup. Alternatively, increase your intake by cooking your soup with plenty of vegetables.
- Reduce portion sizes of starchy foods that are eaten, as this can be quite substantial in the typical West African diet. For instance, if plantain is to be served with a rice dish, reduce your portion of rice.
- Reduce or avoid adding fat and oil to starchy foods.
- Avoid soaking peeled root vegetables like yam, cassava and sweet potatoes for prolonged periods prior to cooking.

Healthy and tasty recipes

With just a few simple changes we can still enjoy many traditional West African dishes as part of a healthy balanced diet. As part of providing proof that the cooking suggestions given actually work, here are few tasty and healthy versions of some popular West African dishes. They are lower in fat and salt than traditional recipes and therefore alright to have most of the time. When your taste buds get used to the lower salt content of these recipes, you may want to consider challenging yourself to go even lower!

Grilled plantain

Serves 2

A popular staple in many West African countries, grilled plantains make a great snack. Closely related to the banana, they are naturally sweet, low in fat and bursting with energy. Served with peanut butter, this recipe is a delicious treat!

Ingredients:

1 large ripe plantain

1 tablespoon reduced-fat peanut butter

Cooking Guide

1. Peel the plantain by chopping both ends off and making a slit along the whole length of its skin. Slide your thumb under the slit to loosen and remove the skin. Cut the plantain in half and then cut each half length-wise. (You should have four pieces altogether).
2. Grill under a medium heat (or chargrill on a barbeque), turning occasionally for about 35 minutes, or until cooked. Cooked plantains are soft inside but not sticky.
3. Serve warm with peanut butter.

Nutritional facts per serving (½ plantain)

Calories 164 kcal; Protein 2.4g; Fat 3g (Saturated Fat 0.6g); Carbohydrate 33.6g; Sugar 7.1g; Fibre 1.7g; Salt 0g

Jollof Rice

Serves 15

Jollof rice is probably the most popular rice dish in West Africa. Though no one knows its origins, it gets its name from the Wolof language where it is known as *benachin* meaning 'one pot'. The vibrant reddish-orange colour makes this dish visually appealing whilst the flavours of all the different ingredients work together to produce the unique taste associated with this dish. Even regional variations cannot dampen the ability of *jollof rice* to tickle everyone's taste buds, making it truly a one-pot dish to relish.

Ingredients:

1 scotch bonnet pepper

1 medium-sized red onion

1 medium-sized white onion

1 cooking spoon (50ml) vegetable oil

4 small stock cubes

1 green sweet pepper

4 medium-sized garlic cloves

1kg basmati rice

1.5 litres water

140g tomato puree

1 tin (400g) plum tomatoes

1 teaspoon ground, dried prawns (crayfish)

1 teaspoon mixed herbs

1 level teaspoon salt

2 bay leaves

Cooking guide

1. Roughly chop the onions and sweet pepper, and puree them in a blender or food processor with 200ml of water, the plum tomatoes, garlic cloves and scotch bonnet pepper.
2. Make a tomato-based sauce by gently heating the oil in a large non-stick saucepan and then adding the pureed tomato, peppers, garlic and onions. Cover and cook over a high heat for about 5 minutes. Add the tomato puree, bay leaves, and stock cubes. Cover and cook for a further 5 minutes, stirring occasionally.
3. Add the mixed herbs and crayfish and cook for a further 5 minutes on a medium heat. Add the remaining water (1.3 litres) and bring to boil.
4. Add the rice, cover and turn down heat. Allow to simmer over a low heat for about 20-25 minutes or until the rice is cooked and tender. During cooking, check and stir occasionally ensuring there is enough liquid to cook the rice so that it does not burn. If there is not enough, make a small well in the middle of the rice and sprinkle a bit of water. Cover and cook till the rice is done.
5. Serve with grilled chicken, fish or meat and brightly coloured steamed vegetables, or a side salad. To save on time, fresh or frozen vegetables can be added to the pan towards the end of cooking, and allowed to steam.

Nutritional facts per serving

Calories 289 kcal; Protein 6.3g; Fat 3.4g (Saturated Fat 0.4g); Carbohydrate 57.6g; Sugar 3.5g; Fibre 0.8g; Salt 0.8g

Okra and dika nut soup

Serves 8

Okra and dika nuts (also known as *ogbono, bobo, andok*) are popular West African soup ingredients and this soup combines the slippery texture of both of them. The slightly bitter aftertaste and spiciness of the dika nuts is complemented beautifully by the sweetness of the onion. As okra is a vegetable, this soup is a great way to reach your 5-a-day target – just don't overcook!

Ingredients:

350g okra

1 small onion

2 tablespoons palm oil

50g dika nut powder

34g tomato puree

850ml water

1 small chicken stock cube

Half a fermented locust bean cake (approx 6g), powdered

3 teaspoons ground, dried prawns (crayfish)

1 level teaspoon salt

120g washed and flaked dried fish

1 scotch bonnet pepper

4 large fresh, white fish fillets (approx 800g)

Cooking Guide

1. Wash the okra and remove stalks. Peel the onion. Roughly chop the okra and onion and puree them together with the scotch bonnet pepper and 200ml of water in a blender or food processor.
2. Gently heat the palm oil in a medium-sized, non-stick saucepan, over a medium heat. Add the dika nut powder and mix well with the oil. Add the tomato puree and mix for about one minute.
3. Add the pureed okra, onion and pepper, stirring for about 5 minutes.
4. Dissolve the stock cube in 300ml of water and add to the saucepan. Add the crayfish and season with salt. Sprinkle in the fermented locust bean powder.
5. Add the remaining water (350ml), the dried fish and the fresh fish fillets. Cover and simmer over a low heat for 15-20 minutes or until the fresh fish is cooked.
6. Serve hot with a starch-based accompaniment such as *pounded yam*, *eba* or *fufu*.

Nutritional facts per serving

Calories 229 kcal; Protein 30.5g; Fat 10.3g (Saturated Fat 2g); Carbohydrate 3.4g; Sugar 2g; Fibre 3.1g; Salt 1.1g

Sunny fruit salad

Serves 6

The vivid colours of this refreshing snack or dessert conjure up childhood memories of sun-drenched days spent growing up in West Africa. Fruit salads are an easy way of reaching your 5-a-day fruit and vegetable target while also getting essential vitamins and minerals. You can adapt this recipe to include other tropical fruit such as banana, guava and papaya – just let your imagination run wild!

Ingredients:

400g just-ripe mango (cubed)

400g watermelon with seeds (cubed)

100g pineapple chunks (fresh or tinned in juice)

Juice and rind of one small lime

1 heaped teaspoon desiccated coconut

Cooking guide

1. Place the mango and watermelon cubes in a bowl with the pineapple chunks.
2. Add the lime juice and rind. Cover and chill in the fridge for about 30-40 minutes.
3. Gently toss the fruit, to mix in the lime juice and rind. Garnish with the desiccated coconut and serve immediately.

Nutritional facts per serving

Calories 71kcal; Protein 0.9g; Fat 0.7g (Saturated Fat 0.5g); Carbohydrate 16.3g; Sugar 16.1g; Fibre 2g; Salt 0g

Steamed bean pudding

Serves 19 as a main dish (38 as an accompaniment)

Steamed bean pudding is a popular West African dish known by a variety of names, including *oleleh* in Sierra Leone and *moin-moin* in Nigeria. An excellent vegetarian dish, it makes a great main dish or can be eaten as an accompaniment. The subtle hint of ginger enhances the taste of this light and fluffy pudding and complements the flavours of all the other ingredients. The bean paste can be prepared and frozen, with the intent of steaming at a later date. Alternatively, it can be steamed and then stored in the freezer, ready for subsequent reheating for a quick meal.

Ingredients

900g dried, pre-peeled black-eyed beans
2 medium onions
3 scotch bonnet peppers (or to taste)
1.75 litres water
50g tomato puree
15 level teaspoons ground, dried prawns (crayfish)
60ml vegetable oil
10g ginger (optional)
3 level teaspoons salt

Cooking method

1. Soak the pre-skinned beans in water to soften. Once softened, puree them with the onions, scotch bonnet peppers, ginger and about 1.4 litres of water, into a smooth paste.

2. Add the tomato puree, crayfish, oil, salt and the rest of the water, to the bean paste. Mix well.
3. Spoon into half-portion (small) takeaway foil containers. (Each container should have 3 cooking spoonfuls of bean paste).
4. Steam for about 30 minutes in a pressure cooker.
5. Serve with bread or with *garri* steeped in cold water.

Nutritional facts per serving (1 foil container)

Calories 197kcal; Protein 11.9g; Fat 3.4g (Saturated Fat 0.6g); Carbohydrate 30.4g; Sugar 2.7g; Fibre 0.9g; Salt 0.8g

Chapter 7

R.S.V.P – Coping With Social Occasions

As West Africans, we love any excuse to party. There's no denying that food brings us together and whatever the occasion, as a community, we celebrate with plenty of food. That's not a bad thing when you consider that our social structure is based on family and community – we just love to be around each other! And where we are, there has to be food in abundance. And don't forget the drinks. At West African functions, there is usually a range of drinks to satisfy even the fussiest of guests.

This strong tradition of sharing is one of the qualities that define our community. It's always about laughter, talking and enjoying each other's company. It's never about how many calories are in the *jollof rice* or how many grams of fat or salt there are in the spicy chicken. As such, there is the tendency to overlook the health consequences of what we are eating - usually food that is salty, high in calories, and high in fat. "What can I do about it, especially as a guest with no control over the catering?" I hear you ask. Until the concept of 'healthy hospitality' catches on (which I hope is very soon), here are some tips to eat healthily on the West African social circuit, and still enjoy yourself:

- Be in control of how much pastry-based snacks, (*chin-chin, puff- puff*, sausage roll, meat pie), you have. Pastry often contains lots of fat and the meat in these products is rarely lean. If you have to indulge, take a small amount and once that's gone, no more.

- Have fruit as a starter instead of pastry, or stick to a low-calorie drink. Eat slowly and focus on the conversation.
- Watch your portions and aim not to pile food onto your plate. You may be surprised at how satisfied you can feel on smaller portions.
- Do take a break of between 10 and 20 minutes before a second helping – it takes this long for your stomach to communicate fullness to your brain!
- Get up and dance. It's a good excuse to have fun and get some physical activity in at the same time.
- Limit how many calories you drink. Malt-based energy drinks like Supermalt and Maltina are laden with glucose and therefore calories. Consider stretching your malt drink by mixing with a diet cola. Remember that non-diet fizzy drinks and alcoholic drinks can also be high in calories.
- Since large portions are usually to be expected, be assertive and ask for smaller portions.
- The fat content of dishes like *ugba* (African oil bean salad) or fried plantain (especially if diced) can be high, so choose or request a smaller portion size or split with a friend or relative.
- Opt for a good-sized serving of salad or vegetables if available. Be sure to watch the dressing if you use any!
- Pace yourself if there are multiple functions to attend over a given time period.
- If available, have fruit after your meal.
- Eat a small snack before attending a social event to take the edge off feeling hungry, and help you stay in control.

- Take the skin off your chicken.
- Stop eating once you're full and don't eat till you are too full.

Eating right at least 80% of the time, when you are fully in control of what you eat, will give you the allowance to relax a little during the 20% of the time when you are not in full control of what you eat - such as at social occasions.

Smart dining out

With life getting busier and busier in our 24-7 world, convenience is king and eating on the go is now quite the norm. The main challenge with eating foods cooked outside your home is the fact that you do not have any control over what goes into your meal during its preparation. Personally, I recommend eating fast food or having takeaways not more than once a month at the most, (twice, if we are really pushing it). In case you're wondering why I'm being so hard-nosed about this, here's why: (a) I believe they are a treat and something to look forward to, but more importantly, (b) these meals tend to be fattier, more calorific and saltier than home-cooked food.

To put this in perspective, at a well-known fast food outlet, a medium or regular-sized burger meal, complete with fries, milk shake and an apple pie for dessert, will supply you with 1485 calories, 80g of sugar, 64g of fat (including 23g of cholesterol-raising saturated fat), and 3.6g of salt. That's almost 75% of the daily calorie allowance for an average-sized woman (2000 calories to be exact). This meal also supplies nearly all the daily fat allowance (70g), and over half the daily salt allowance (6g), of an average-sized woman - in just one meal! Deciding to go 'large' brings the grand total of just one meal to a whopping 1735 calories, 74g of fat (including 25g of saturated fat) and 4g of salt!! Is this really value for money?

It's a similar story for child-sized meals - even the value added by a free toy cannot hide the fact that this sort of meal should be eaten occasionally.

Fast food outlets are not the only culprits – nice, sit down restaurants with a lovely ambience can be just as guilty. Don't get me wrong, eating out at your favourite restaurant is fine and should be a social and enjoyable experience. Variety is the spice of life after all, and we (especially the ladies or whoever cooks most of the meals at home), all need a break from being in the kitchen sometimes. Nevertheless, unless the menu clearly states that the restaurant consciously uses healthier recipes or cooking methods, then chances are that your meal will be high in fat (and therefore calories), salt, and in some cases, sugar.

We also need to consider the issue of generous or large portions that as consumers we associate with getting good value for money. Many restaurants use large portion sizes to convey the fact that they are listening to our demands, so as to encourage and retain our patronage.

Making better choices when eating out

So how can you get round the potential threat posed to your health by eating outside your home? Remember that eating out is an enjoyable part of life and that modest amounts of high calorie foods can be eaten without any detriment to your health, if eaten occasionally. The trick is to consciously make as a good a choice as possible by balancing higher fat choices with lower fat ones. So for example, if you choose a high fat main dish, then choose a lower fat starter and lower fat dessert. In the next section I have suggested a few pointers to help you make better choices from the menu, regardless of the cuisine.

West African restaurants

West African cuisine is known for its emphasis on starchy foods, and generous portion sizes feature at many West African restaurants. So, in addition to the tips given for coping at special occasions:

- Ask for a smaller portion when placing your order or request a 'take away' container to take some off before you start to eat.
- Make better choices such as choosing grilled meat e.g. *suya* or grilled fish rather than fried versions.
- Request a side dish to skim oil off dishes with an oily layer.
- Be assertive and find out how a dish is prepared prior to ordering, or request that your meal is prepared to your (healthier) requirements.
- Eat small portions of high fat dishes like *ugba* (African oil bean salad) or fried plantain.

Chinese cuisine

Traditional Chinese cuisine is based on steamed rice, fresh vegetables and fish which are all low in fat. It also favours stir-frying, which is a great way to cook foods, especially when less fat is used. This method of cooking preserves both the flavour, and the nutritional quality of fresh vegetables. These healthy qualities have been lost in a bid to cater for the Western palate, and most Chinese restaurants place a greater emphasis on meat and fried foods.

Choose:

- Clear soups, such as won-ton or hot and sour soups.
- Stir-fried dishes, such as beef and pepper or chicken and pineapple.
- Steamed or boiled rice or noodles.

- Steamed or stir-fried vegetables.
- Steamed dim sum. Some types of dim sum are deep-fried or have hot fat or lard poured over them.
- Dishes based on soy sauce, chilli or oyster sauces - such as beef in black bean sauce, and vegetable or tofu dishes in soy sauce. However, check that the tofu has not been deep-fried first.
- Lychees or other fruit for dessert.

Avoid or have small portions of:

- Fried starters e.g. spring rolls, prawn crackers, egg rolls and fried won-tons.
- Syrup-based dishes e.g. sticky spare ribs and sweet and sour dishes.
- Fried rice or noodles.
- Meat or vegetables cooked in batter or deep-fried e.g. crispy fried beef or duck and crispy seaweed.
- Dim sum which has not been steamed.
- Dishes containing battered and fried meat e.g. sweet and sour pork or chicken in lemon sauce.
- Fruit fritters or deep-fried ice-cream.

If your dish is being prepared to order, ask the restaurant to use less fat, salt and sugar. Dishes based on vegetables tend to be lower in fat, so make the most of these and be aware that meat or chicken dishes containing nuts can be high in calories.

Italian cuisine

Pasta and pizza are well-known dishes featuring in Italian-themed restaurants. However, both can have a very high fat content - even pizza with low-fat toppings. Salads are popular in these restaurants so base your meal on this and share a pizza with a friend. Be aware that some sauces served with pasta may contain a lot of fat.

Choose:

- Vegetable-based soups (such as minestrone) as a starter. You can have this with plain crusty bread or grissini (breadsticks).
- Grated vegetables or salads with a low fat dressing (or no dressing).
- Tomato or vegetable sauces, (such as napoli, arrabiata or Bolognese), to accompany any type of pasta.
- Stone-baked pizzas, as they are typically lower in fat. Likewise, regular or thick base pizzas are better than thin base ones.
- Lean meat and vegetable toppings such as ham, tuna, prawns, pepper, pineapple, sweetcorn, mushrooms, tomato, onion, green pepper or chilli.
- Sorbets as a dessert.

Avoid or have small portions of:

- Garlic bread, particularly if it has a cheesy topping.
- Antipasto i.e. salami or vegetables in oil.
- Creamy or cheese-based sauces and dishes based on them, e.g. cannelloni, lasagne or carbonara dishes.
- Pesto and high fat dressings like mayonnaise.

- Pizzas cooked with added oil and stuffed pizza bases e.g. stuffed with cheese.
- High-fat pizza toppings such as salami, pepperoni, extra cheese, olives.
- Extra cheese on pasta dishes.

Fast Food Outlets

Fast food places offer a variety of quick, relatively inexpensive and highly convenient food. Generally these foods tend to be fried and therefore high in fat and calories. Choosing small or medium portions instead of large can help reduce your calorie intake.

Choose:

- Plain chicken, fish, beef and vegetarian burgers.
- Wholemeal buns if available.
- Salad or chopped vegetables.
- Fruit and low-fat yoghurt.
- Fruit juice, diet soft drinks and water.

Avoid or have smaller portions of:

- Burgers with added cheese or high fat dressings such as mayonnaise, as they can contain up to three times as much fat as a plain burger.
- Deep-fried foods such as chicken nuggets, chicken in batter and fish burgers, as they are high in fat.
- Coleslaw.
- Ice cream and similar desserts.
- Thick milk shakes, as they can contain up to 45g of sugar and 6g of fat.
- Doughnuts, pies and muffins, all of which are high in fat and sugar.

Middle Eastern cuisine

Cuisine from the Middle East is known for its subtle flavours from aromatic spices and herbs such as mint and parsley. It is also known for its generous use of olive oil which although healthy, can result in high calorie dishes.

Choose:

- Flat breads such as pitta.
- Shish kebab or souvlaki made with lean meat and skinless poultry.
- Dips like hummus, taramasalata and tabouli. Ask about their oil content though.
- Salads.
- Dolmades and cabbage rolls.
- Tzatziki (yogurt and cucumber dip).
- Sweets without fat such as Turkish delight.

Avoid or have smaller portions of:

- Fried dishes like fried aubergine (eggplant).
- Moussaka and other meat dishes with sauces.
- Shawarma or doner kebab.
- Couscous, as restaurant versions can be very high in fat.
- Olive oil-based dips and tahini-based dips e.g. baba ganoush.
- Extra olive oil drizzled over dishes.
- Pastries such as baklava and other high-fat desserts such as halva.

Tex-mex and Mexican cuisine

Tex-mex and Mexican cuisine is based on rice and beans, which in moderation are fine. However, fried dishes feature as part of the cuisine and choosing high fat sauces and dressings can further increase the fat content of dishes.

Choose:

- Fish, chicken or vegetables as fillings for fajitas.
- Salsa (tomato and chilli dip), frijoles (bean dip) and tomato-based sauces.
- Soft flour or corn tortillas.
- Salad, vegetables and fruit.
- Grilled fish or chicken.

Avoid or have small portions of:

- Enchiladas, tacos and burritos.
- Fried dishes, such as refried beans, fried enchiladas, fried potatoes.
- Dishes with added cheese.
- Sour cream.
- High calorie dressings
- Guacamole.

Thai cuisine

Infused with flavour from lemon grass, garlic and a host of other spices and condiments, Thai cuisine has a number of healthy options, as it is based on steamed rice, vegetables and fish.

Choose:

- Clear soups containing noodles, vegetables and meat.

- Stir-fried chicken or vegetables.
- Bean curd (tofu).
- Meat dishes cooked with chilli, lemon grass or soy sauce.
- Plain steamed rice or noodles.
- Salad or vegetables.
- Fruit for dessert.

Avoid or have small portions of:

- Satay (peanut-based) sauces.
- Curries with cream or coconut milk.
- Coconut rice, sticky rice, fried rice or fried noodles.
- Spring rolls and fish cakes.
- Desserts such as coconut ice-cream, deep-fried bananas and traditional Thai sweets.

Indian cuisine

Traditional Indian cuisine is high in high fibre as dishes are based on pulses, vegetables and rice. However, many Indian restaurants use fatty meats in dishes and add more fat during cooking, resulting in high fat dishes. As most sauces may have a lot of fat, savour the flavour of a dish by eating the meat and vegetables and leaving the high fat sauce.

Choose:

- Drier or baked dishes such as tandoori, tikka, karia or bhuna dishes cooked without sugar or fat.
- High-fibre, lentil-based dishes, such as dahl and dhansaak.
- Plain green salads.

- Boiled or steamed rice.
- Indian breads (e.g. chapatti, grilled poppadoms, plain naan bread, or tandoori roti), made without added fat.
- Vegetable curries e.g. saag (spinach), aloo gobi (cabbage), made without cream or ghee.
- Meat curries with a tomato base such as jalfrezi and balti.
- Yogurt-based meat dishes.

Avoid or have small portions of:

- Fried starters such as bhajis, pakoras, parathas, puris, deep-fried poppadoms and samosas.
- Dishes containing ghee (clarified butter), such as madras, vindaloo and dupiaza.
- Meat curries, as they tend to be based on fatty meats.
- Pasandas, masalas and kormas.
- Rice dishes with added fat like pilau, biryani and fried rice.

Sandwich bars

Low-fat fillings are available in many sandwich bars and while bread is a good carbohydrate source, bear in mind that some breads may have added fat.

Choose:

- Granary or wholemeal bread or rolls.
- Low-fat spread instead of butter, or ask for spreads to be used sparingly.
- Lower fat fillings such as ham, chicken, egg, tuna or cottage cheese.

- Low-fat natural yoghurt makes a good alternative dressing to mayonnaise.
- Salad or grated vegetables as part of your sandwich.

Avoid or have small portions of:

- High fat dressings such as mayonnaise and salad cream, or request low calorie versions.
- High-fat fillings, like sausage or bacon (as they tend to be fried), and full fat cheese which is sometimes mixed with mayonnaise.

Fish and chip shops

Traditionally seen as the quintessential British dish, fish and chips is a popular takeaway meal of deep-fried potatoes and fish in batter. A variety of other foods are available at fish and chip shops, but like fish and chips, they tend to be fried or high in fat so you need to choose carefully.

Choose:

- Fish, but eat only the fish and leave the batter.
- Potato wedges or thick cut chips as they absorb less oil during frying.
- Smaller portions of chips, or share with a friend.
- Side salads or vegetables.
- Kebabs based on lean meats e.g. shish kebabs (made from lamb), or chicken. Have small or medium portions.

Avoid or have small portions of:

- High-fat processed foods, such as saveloys, pies and fried sausages.
- High-fat dressings and sauces like mayonnaise.

- Deep-fried meats and doner or kofta kebabs.

Pubs and restaurants

Nowadays in the UK, there are healthy eating options on the menus at many pubs and restaurants. If this is not the case at your chosen restaurant or pub, then base your meal on starchy foods (such as breads, baked or boiled potatoes, pasta or rice), with a moderate portion of chicken, fish or beans. Finally, bring balance to your meal by including some salad or vegetables.

Choose:

- Potato dishes not cooked with fat - jacket, boiled or new potatoes, instead of chips.
- Low-fat fillings such as baked beans, cottage cheese, tuna, chicken or vegetables.
- Tomato-based sauces for pasta.
- Sorbet, fruit salad, fresh fruit, or jelly for dessert. Alternatively, you don't have to have a dessert.
- Semi-skimmed milk in teas and coffees.
- Fruit-based starters, consommé or vegetable soup, shellfish (without dressing), grilled fish, or smoked salmon.
- A la carte and avoid buffets.
- Plenty of vegetables - without a coating of butter or a rich creamy sauce. Or choose a side salad (without the dressing), and a roll. Use margarine or low-fat spread instead of butter in your roll.

Avoid or have small portions of:

- Pastries, tarts, chocolate gateaux and cheesecakes. These are all high in fat and sugar, so only indulge on very special occasions.

- High fat starters such as deep-fried foods, pate, egg mayonnaise, creamy soups or dips.
- Mayonnaise-rich foods for example, coleslaw, tuna mayonnaise, and chicken mayonnaise.
- Fried foods and pastry items as a main course.
- Creamy or high fat dressings and sauces.
- Coffee with cream.
- Jacket potatoes with margarine, butter, or high fat cheese (e.g. ched-dar).

Alcohol

Special occasions and eating out can often mean consuming some form of alcohol as part of the meal. Alcohol is made from the fermentation of sugars present in starchy foods such as grains and cereals. It can be part of a healthy eating plan,

Measuring your alcohol intake

In the UK, the unit system is used to quantify the amount of alcohol consumed. Units take into account the amount of alcohol in a certain amount of alcoholic drink. Known as Alcohol by Volume, or ABV, this is shown as a number with a percent sign on the bottle i.e. 4%ABV. One standard unit in the UK is the equivalent of:

- Half a pint of lager, cider or beer (285ml) 3.5% ABV
- A small glass of wine (125ml) 9% ABV
- One shot or pub measure of spirits (25ml) 40% ABV

as long as it is drunk sensibly and in moderation, within the guidelines set by the relevant health authorities.

From a nutritional perspective, alcohol has no nutrients to offer, just calories. One gram of alcohol contains seven calories (7kcals), making it the next most energy dense substance after fat (which has 9kcals per gram). Additionally, drinking alcohol tends to lower your resolve to make informed food choices. This can lead to unhealthy food choices and overeating, so it's really important to stay in control to avoid literally pouring on the pounds.

And just in case you're wondering whether you misheard that alcohol is supposed to be good for you, there is some evidence that red wine can be beneficial in the prevention of stroke and heart disease, due to its content of polyphenols and flavanoids – two antioxidants that can help fight free-radicals. However, the studies show that this is more applicable to men over the age of 40, and women after the menopause, which is when there is increased risk of developing heart disease.

It is important to note that information on what constitutes a unit is not available for all alcoholic drinks. Consequently, it is easy to drink more than the recommended number of units in just one sitting without even realising. This would certainly apply to favourite beers and lagers brewed and enjoyed in many West African countries, and which are also available around the world. The table below shows how many units are in a bottle of some popular West African beers:

Country	Beer	Volume	ABV	Units
Benin Republic	La Beninoise	630ml	4.9%	3
Burkina Faso	Biere du Burkina	650ml	4.2%	2.7
	SOB.B.BRA	650ml	4.2%	2.7

Country	Beer	Volume	ABV	Units
Cameroon	Castel beer	330ml	5.2%	1.7
	Beaufort	650ml	4.6%	3
	Beaufort 6.9	330ml	6.9%	2.3
	Millennium	650ml	5%	3.2
Gabon	Regab	650ml	4.5%	3
Gambia	Julbrew regular	280ml	4.7%	1.3
	Julbrew export	330ml	5.5%	1.8
	Julbrew strong	280ml	7.5%	2
	Julbrew very strong	280ml	10%	2.8
Ghana	Club	625ml	5%	3
	Gulder	625ml	5%	3
	Star lager	625ml	5%	3
	Stone strong lager	625ml	5.7%	3.6
	Castle Milk Stout	625ml	6%	3.7
Guinea-Bissau	Pampa	500ml	5.1%	2.5
Ivory Coast	Bock	330ml	4.6%	1.5
	Mamba lager	659ml	5.2%	3.4
Nigeria	Gulder	600ml	5.2%	3
	Guinness	330ml	7.5%	2.5
	Star lager	600ml	5%	3
	Legend Stout	300ml	7.5%	2.2
Senegal	Biere La Gazelle	630ml	4.2%	2.6
Togo	Eku Bavaria	330ml	5.4%	1.8
	Flag Spéciale	650ml	5.2%	3.3

You can calculate the number of units in any alcoholic drink using this formula:

Strength (ABV) x Volume (ml) ÷ 1000 = No. of units.

Enjoying alcohol sensibly

- For every alcoholic drink you have, aim to have a non-alcoholic one, preferably a diet or low-calorie version, or water. This way, you can slash your total alcohol intake in half.

- Per day, women should have no more than 1-2 units and men no more than 2-3 units. Men have a slightly larger alcohol allowance than women because of the difference in body composition – they tend to have less body fat than women and so are able to process alcohol more efficiently.
- Spread your units out over the week, allowing for some alcohol-free days. Saving your recommended alcohol units for the weekend is classified as binge drinking.
- If losing weight is on your agenda, alcohol intake should be limited even more, especially as it is high in calories. Furthermore, over-indulging on alcohol can impair your ability to make better food choices and stay in control.
- Select light versions of alcoholic drinks where possible. "Light" means fewer calories, so these products are not calorie- or alcohol-free. As such you still need to limit your intake.
- Keep water available to quench your thirst while you drink alcoholic beverages.
- Learn to sip your drink to make it last longer.

Chapter 8

Shopping For Health

Believe it or not, most of our health choices are made whilst we are doing our food shopping. Whether you shop at a supermarket, cash and carry, or market, each time you put something into your shopping trolley, you're making a decision that will either negatively or positively affect your health and that of your family. Think back to your last shopping trip. What did your shopping trolley look like? Did you pay any attention to the food labels on what you put in?

Whenever I've spoken on healthy diet and lifestyle, the topic of understanding food labels never fails to grab (and hold) the attention of the audience. Not surprising, when you consider that research in the UK suggests that almost 6 in 10 adults experience difficulty working out if a food is healthy by looking at its packaging or label. Being 'label-savvy' can make the difference between literally paying for ill health and avoiding it in the first place. So what's in a food label and how can it help with your health?

Food labels are the means by which food manufacturers and retailers communicate information about a food product to us. They provide the information you need to compare similar products and enable you to make an informed choice between the so many products that confront you in the supermarket. By UK law, two pieces of information must be on a food label: firstly, the ingredients, listed in order of descending weight, and secondly, nutrition information about the product. Nutrition information is provided per 100g for total calories, fat, saturated fat, sugar, salt (or sodium) and fibre, as well as per serving. The 'per 100g' information enables you to compare one product with another, whilst the 'per serving' information tells you how much of each nutrient is present in a suggested serving. The nutrient content per serving is also expressed as a percentage of the average recommended daily intake or guideline daily amount (GDA). Usually on the front of the packaging, it will read something like this '...provides 20% of your guideline daily amount for salt'.

In the UK, to make things even easier, some food manufacturers and retailers have also adopted the multiple traffic light system for their front-of-package labelling. Nutrients are colour-coded to indicate the amounts in one serving compared to recommended amounts i.e. red for high, amber for medium, and green for low. With this system, you are looking for foods with green for most nutrients; foods with red for most nutrients should be eaten occasionally and in smaller quantities.

Take a look at a few labels. You'll notice that foods that are often high in sugar tend to be low in fat and vice versa. This is known as the fat-sugar see-saw, as both fat and sugar make foods taste good. Unfortunately, too much of either is bad for you which is why foods containing these should be eaten occasionally.

Label reading - The highs and lows

Look at the 'per 100g' column of a food label and compare it with the table on the next page. If for example, total fat is 8g per 100g, then it is a medium fat product because 8g is between 3g and 20g. Similarly, 3g or less is low fat, while 20g or more is high fat.

Per 100g	Total fat	Saturated fat	Sugar	Salt (Sodium)	Fibre
Low	3g	1.5g	2g	0.25g (0.1g)	0.5g
High	20g	5g	10g	1.25g (0.5g)	3g

So how do your current food choices measure up? Apart from fibre, foods that are high in the other nutrients should be eaten occasionally. Reading food labels may initially lengthen your shopping trip, but with practice you'll soon become proficient. Your health will certainly thank you for it.

Label reading 101

- Ingredients are listed by amount starting from the greatest to the least. So if sugar, for example, is among the first four ingredients, then that product has a high sugar content.
- Nutrition information 'per 100g' enables you compare one brand of say, bread with another, because it provides a standardised fig-ure.
- Nutrition information 'per serving' or portion shows you how much salt, sugar, fat etc, is present in a portion, as stipulated by a manufacturer.
- For foods you eat regularly, check the 'per serving' column; for those you eat occasionally check the 'per 100g' column.
- What the manufacturer considers to be a portion or serving can sometimes be unrealistic, making it very easy to consume more calories than needed.
- Products with low lower fat, sugar and salt content are better choices.

- Guideline Daily Amounts (GDAs) give an indication of how much an average-sized man, woman and child should have in terms of calories and nutrients, and show how much a portion of a particular food will contribute to those amounts e.g. '*... provides 16% of your GDA for calcium*'.
- With the multiple traffic light labelling system, you are looking to choose foods that are mainly green for the different nutrients, reserving mainly reds for occasional use.

Ten Handy Shopping Tips

1. **Plan, plan, plan.** Planning before you head off to the supermarket will help you shop more economically, so be organised and shop from a list. Organisation is an investment – you need to invest time to create or save time.
2. **Bulk-buy** from specialist cash and carry warehouses, warehouse clubs or super stores, and share with friends or family. Be aware that membership may be required. Shopping at specialist markets for meat, fish and fruit and vegetables also represents good value for money. The only downside is likely to be the early morning trip, as most specialist markets start in the early hours of the morning!
3. **Buy lean.** For meats, buy as lean as you can afford, as it's better value for money and better for your health. Ask your butcher to remove fat from meat and take the skin off poultry – after all, you are paying for the service.
4. **Buy in season.** Fresh fruit and vegetables in season tend to be tastier, contain more nutrients and are better value for money. Frozen fruit and vege-

tables are just as good as fresh and also represent good value for money. Frozen corn on the cob can be cooked in the microwave without the hassle of de-husking the cobs yourself.

5. **Supermarket-own brands can be just as good.** Don't be afraid to experiment. Depending on the product, supermarket-own brands can be just as good as or even better than leading brands, both from a taste and nutrition perspective.
6. **Take advantage of special offers, coupons and money off vouchers**, but only buy what you need and will use. Remember that a bargain is only a bargain if you need it.
7. **Don't fall for marketing strategies.** My favourite one is 'cholesterol-free' vegetable oil. There is nothing special about cholesterol-free vegetable oils as vegetable oils do not contain cholesterol anyway. Also, olive oil has proven health benefits, but can be expensive. A much cheaper alternative is rapeseed oil which is usually sold as vegetable oil in most UK supermarkets. Rapeseed oil has a similar profile to olive oil and confers the same health benefits!
8. **Shop at reputable African food shops to prevent food safety issues,** (including dermestes beetle infestation in dried fish, salmonella and aflatoxin contamination in melon seeds (*egusi, akatsewa*) and dika nuts (*apon, ogbono*), as well as aflatoxin contamination in peanut products). This is especially important if you run a catering business. In the UK, random checks are made on imported foods and there are set limits for what is considered safe. Shopping at reputable shops also ensures that you get what you pay for. For example, in the UK, mutton is often incorrectly (and sometimes unscrupulously) marketed as goat meat.

9. **P for pulses, P for protein.** Pulses such as beans are cheaper than meat, and are a great protein source. Use them to stretch meat dishes or for meat-free days without losing any protein. They are also a great source of fibre.
10. **Never shop on empty.** Supermarkets fully understand the effect that the smell of freshly baked bread has on shoppers, so they pipe it through the store. One whiff of this aroma on an empty stomach is enough to send even the most resolute shopper into a complete shopping frenzy.

Appendices

Appendix 1: Nutrients in West African Foods at a Glance

Nutrients	RNI	Functions	Sources
Vitamin A (Retinol)	Men 700mcg Women 600mcg	Essential for good vision, especially night vision, normal bone growth, reproduction, skin health and mucous membrane health.	Vitamin A is found pre-formed in foods of animal origin such as liver, West African giant snails, fish liver oils, eggs and dairy products such as cheese and milk. Retinol is also found in non-animal sources in the form of beta-carotene which is converted into vitamin A by the body. Rich sources of beta-carotene include: palm oil, palm fruit, pumpkin, watermelon, plantain, carrot, guava, ripe mango, okra, yellow corn, sweet peppers, banana, African pear, ripe papaya, yellow varieties of yam, sweet potato (yellow- or orange-coloured), garden eggs, red scotch bonnet peppers, bird peppers and a wide variety of leafy green vegetables including baobab leaves, horseradish tree leaves, red sorrel, cowpea leaves, sweet potato leaves, cassava leaves, tamarind tree leaves, bush okra leaves, pumpkin leaves, African spinach, bitterleaf, red sorrel, Lagos spinach, fluted pumpkin leaves, waterleaf.

Nutrients	RNI	Functions	Sources
Vitamin B_1 (Thiamin)	Men 1.0mg Women 0.8mg	Helps the body convert fats and carbohydrates into energy. Needed for normal growth and development and for the proper functioning of heart and nervous and digestive systems.	Soya beans, liver, beef, pork, fermented foods (e.g. fermented starchy gruels and doughs, fermented locust beans), garden eggs, red sorrel, egusi seeds, groundnuts, sesame seeds, African pear, pineapple, avocado, palm wine, black-eyed beans and other pulses, rice, African pepper, African nutmeg, edible insects.
Vitamin B_2 (Riboflavin)	Men 1.3mg Women 1.1mg	Essential for the release of energy from carbohydrates and for normal growth and development. Protects the nervous system and helps in the storage of glucose in the body in the form of glycogen.	African spinach, okra, eggs, meat, fish, fermented foods (fermented locust beans, fermented African oil bean, fermented castor seeds (ogiri Igbo), fermented starchy gruels), milk and dairy products, meat, garden eggs, African pear , red sorrel, sweet potato leaves, egusi seeds, sesame seeds, pineapple, avocado, palm wine, black-eyed beans and other pulses, African pepper, African nutmeg, edible insects.
Vitamin B_3 (Niacin)	Men 17mg Women 13mg	Needed for the utilisation of energy from food.	Red sorrel, egusi seeds, groundnuts, sesame seeds, fermented locust beans, mango, African pear, avocado, palm wine, guinea fowl, black-eyed beans and other pulses, rice, African pepper, African nutmeg.
Vitamin B_6 (Pyridoxine)	Men 1.4mcg Women 1.2mcg	Needed for the metabolism of amino acids and the formation of haemoglobin.	Groundnuts, ginger, banana, palm wine, meat and poultry (guinea fowl, chicken, turkey), yam.

Nutrients	RNI	Functions	Sources
Vitamin B_{12}	Men 1.5mcg Women 1.5mcg	Needed for normal growth and development and for the production of red blood cells. It is needed for the functioning of the nervous system.	Palm wine, dairy products, offal (kidneys, heart and liver), beef, eggs, seafood, fermented starchy gruels, garden eggs, guinea fowl, fresh and dried prawns, crayfish.
Folic acid	Men 200mcg Women 200mcg (400mcg if planning a baby and through first 12 weeks of pregnancy).	Plays a vital role in the production of new cells and is needed for normal growth and development. Used by body to make haemoglobin, an important part of red blood cells.	Black-eyed beans and other pulses, groundnuts, banana, oranges and orange juice, African pear, avocado, liver, kidney, eggs, early season yams, corn, dark green leafy vegetables such as fluted pumpkin leaves, African spinach, African joint fir leaves, sweet potato leaves, cassava leaves.
Vitamin C	Men 40mg Women 40mg	Essential for the formation of collagen, a structural protein in the body that strengthens bones and blood vessels as well as anchors teeth in gums. Vital for growth, tissue repair and wound healing. Has antioxidant properties and enhances iron absorption from the intestines.	Baobab fruit, cabbage, cashew apple, oranges, lemons and limes, guava, mango, watermelon, ripe papaya, banana, pineapple, sweet peppers (red and orange-coloured), sweet potato (yellow- or orange-coloured), tomato, fluted pumpkin leaves, Lagos spinach, African spinach, red sorrel, African star apple, plantain, cassava, tiger nuts, garden eggs, bitterleaf, sweet potato leaves, cassava leaves, bush okra leaves, African joint fir leaves, okra, red scotch bonnet peppers, red bird peppers, cloves, velvet tamarind, mango, African pear, sugarcane, corn, African pepper, African nutmeg.

Nutrients	RNI	Functions	Sources
Vitamin D	None set in the UK	Plays a vital role In the absorption and use of calcium and phosphorus. Important in the formation and health of teeth, bones and cartilage.	Oily fish (mackerel, west African herring, West African sardines, salmon, tuna, sardines), egg yolk, sunlight on exposed skin.
Vitamin E	None set in the UK	Has powerful antioxidant properties protecting the body against damage from free radicals. Helps make red blood cells and prevents blood from clotting and protects vitamin A from chemical changes.	Fermented locust beans, fermented egusi seeds (ogiri), green leafy vegetables, groundnuts, meat, groundnut oil, soya beans, palm oil, palm fruit, tiger nuts, coconut, sesame seeds, mango, African pear, avocado, soya oil, sesame oil, coconut oil, tiger nut oil.
Vitamin K	None set in the UK	Required for normal blood clotting.	Green leafy vegetables such as fluted pumpkin leaves, Lagos spinach, African spinach, red sorrel, bitterleaf, sweet potato leaves, cassava leaves, bush okra leaves and African joint fir leaves; cloves, African pear, banana, avocado.

Nutrients	RNI	Functions	Sources
Calcium	Men 700mg Women 700mg	Needed for blood clotting, muscle contraction and nerve signals	Fresh and dried leafy vegetables such as fluted pumpkin, African spinach, baobab leaves, bush okra, Lagos spinach, red sorrel leaves, African pear; baobab fruit, cassava, milk and milk products, calcium-enriched milk substitutes, soft bones from fish and meats, indigenous rock salt , okra, millet, plantain, garri, cocoyam, garden eggs, egusi seeds, dika nuts, sesame seeds, African pepper, African nutmeg, Ashanti pepper, melegueta pepper, African mahogany seeds, cloves, spicy cedar seeds, African nut seeds, African star apples, watermelon, sugar cane, banana, papaya, West African giant snails, dried prawns and shrimps, stockfish, black-eyed beans and other pulses, rice, wild basil, fermented egusi seeds (ogiri), horse eye beans.
Potassium	Men 3500mg Women 3500mg	Controls the amount of water and maintains the correct pH balance in the body.	Banana, African star apples , tomatoes, oranges, avocado, baobab seeds, yam, cassava, sweet potato, watermelon, okra, mango, papaya, coconut, plantain, tiger nuts, African pear, garden eggs, fluted pumpkin leaves, baobab leaves, egusi seeds, dika nuts, coconut, African pepper, aidan fruit pod seeds, dairy products, meat, bird peppers, African pepper, African nutmeg, ginger, horse eye beans, cola nuts, West African giant snails, dried and fresh prawns, fonio, wild basil, fermented egusi seeds (ogiri).

Nutrients	RNI	Functions	Sources
Iron	Men 8.7mg Women 14.8mg	Major component of the red pigment, haemoglobin in blood, which carries oxygen round the body.	Beans, groundnuts, African star apples, shellfish (fresh and dried prawns and shrimps), dried fish, West African giant snails, egusi seeds, sesame seeds, egg yolk, okra seeds, plantain, groundnuts, offal (kidney, liver, heart), meat, poultry, soya beans, black-eyed beans and other pulses, fresh and dried green leafy vegetables e.g. fluted pumpkin, African spinach, bush okra leaves, bitterleaf, red sorrel, baobab leaves, African joint fir leaves, Lagos spinach; cocoyam, garden eggs, African pepper, aidan fruit pod seeds, red scotch bonnet peppers, bird peppers, African nutmeg, African pepper, melegueta pepper, African mahogany seeds, cloves, sugar cane, banana, papaya, avocado, guinea fowl, African giant snails, tropical periwinkles, stockfish, black-eyed beans and other pulses, rice, fermented egusi seeds (ogiri), edible insects, horse eye beans.
Copper	Men 1.2mg Women 1.2mg	Production of pigment in hair, eyes and skin, development of healthy teeth and bones. Also has antioxidant properties.	Seafood (crab, lobster, tropical oysters), sesame seeds, liver, almonds, African spinach, fluted pumpkin leaves, groundnuts, African nutmeg, ginger, African star apples, avocado, fermented egusi seeds (ogiri), edible insects.

Nutrients	RNI	Functions	Sources
Magnesium	Men 300mg Women 270mg	Plays a vital role in bone and teeth formation and is involved in transmitting nerve signals	Dried leafy vegetables, African plum, African spinach, okra, egusi seeds, coconut, meat, nuts (cashew and peanuts), cocoyam, sorghum, black-eyed beans and other pulses, palm fruit, African pepper, aidan fruit pod seeds, red scotch bonnet peppers, bird peppers, ginger, cloves, African star apples, watermelon, banana, papaya, West African giant snails, dried and fresh prawns, corn, wild basil, fermented egusi seeds (ogiri), horse eye beans.
Selenium	Men 75mcg Women 60mcg	Normal functioning of the immune system and thyroid gland. It also has antioxidant properties which protect cells from free radical damage.	Mackerel, shellfish (tropical oysters, tropical periwinkles dried and fresh prawns), fish, poultry, bitterleaf, black-eyed beans and other pulses.
Zinc	Men 9.5mg Women 7mg	Needed for normal cell division, growth and repair; maintaining a healthy immune system and for wound healing.	Meat, offal, fish, poultry, edible insects, egusi seeds, sesame seeds, West African giant snails, cereals, groundnuts, crab, oysters, eggs, dairy products, black-eyed beans and other pulses, African star apples, banana, fluted pumpkin leaves, African spinach, baobab leaves, African pepper, African nutmeg, African mahogany seeds, papaya, avocado, fresh and dried prawns, corn, fermented egusi seeds (ogiri).

Nutrients	RNI	Functions	Sources
Sodium	Men 1600mg Women 1600mg	Necessary for maintaining water balance in the body as well as muscle and nerve activity.	Baobab leaves, African pepper, African nutmeg, West African giant snails, dried and fresh prawns, fermented egusi seeds (ogiri), indigenous rock salt, table salt, indigenous salts from the ashes of tree barks (potash).
Sulphur	None set for the UK	Needed for a number of body functions, including making amino acids and the hormone, insulin.	Egusi seeds, leafy green vegetables, dairy products, meat, offal, egg yolks, black-eyed beans and other pulses, nuts, seafood such as dried and fresh prawns, tropical periwinkles.
Manganese	None set for the UK	Needed for the proper functioning of enzymes.	Baobab leaves, egusi seeds, groundnuts, African nutmeg, ginger, cloves, pineapple, black-eyed beans, tea, pepper fruit, onions, garlic, tea, African pepper, Ashanti pepper, ginger, cloves, wild basil, African pepper, African nutmeg, melegueta pepper, garlic, dried aidan tree fruit, country onions.

Nutrients	RNI	Functions	Sources
Phosphorus	Men 550mg Women 550mg	Essential for the formation of bones and teeth.	African pear, African spinach, fish, cereals, egusi seeds, groundnuts, dika nuts, soft bones from fish and meats, meat, seafood (e.g. tropical periwinkles), baobab seeds, plantain, cassava, garri, cocoyam, tiger nuts, bitterleaf, baobab leaves, coconut, African pepper, African nutmeg, Ashanti pepper, melegueta pepper, African mahogany seeds, spicy cedar seeds, African star apples, watermelon, papaya, avocado, cola nuts, West African giant snails, prawns (fresh and dried), fonio, black-eyed beans and other pulses, fermented egusi seeds (ogiri), rice.
Phytochemicals (Phenols, polyphenols, flavanoids, tannins, saponins, lycopene, organosulphides, phytoes-trogens).		Exert a protective effect against free radical damage due their antioxidant properties.	Dried and fresh leafy vegetables, soya beans, beta-carotene containing foods (see sources of vitamin A); spices and herbs like pepper fruit, onions, garlic, tea, African pepper, Ashanti pepper, ginger, cloves, wild basil, African nutmeg, melegueta pepper, tomatoes, bird peppers, aidan tree fruit and seeds, scotch bonnet pepper, country onion.

Appendix 2: Healthy Haircare for an Active Lifestyle

You can prevent sweat damage to your hair during exercise by controlling moisture and salt build-up. Salty build-up causes hair breakage, shedding, dullness, and dryness. Speak with your stylist or hairdresser regarding an appropriate regime to manage your hair – a regime which takes into consideration your budget and active lifestyle. Remember that healthy hair is hair that is cared for and can be natural, relaxed or braided. Here are some tips to care for your hair, whatever your hairstyle:

Natural hair

- Use a moisturising conditioner or hot oil treatment to condition your hair every week.
- Apply a light conditioning oil to your hair and scalp every day.
- Protect your hair each time you swim with a swimming cap. If you do not use a cap, remember to shampoo or use a cream rinse after every swimming session.
- If you have a close-cropped style, trim your hair every 4 to 6 weeks.

Relaxed hair

Chemical relaxers make your hair fragile so you need to treat relaxed hair with extra care.

- Use a wide-toothed comb to style your hair.
- Trim your hair every 6 to 8 weeks to keep your hairstyle in shape.
- As hair grows faster in warm weather, you're likely to need more frequent touch-ups to your roots during warm months than during cold months. Always speak with your hairdresser to ensure adequate time is allowed between touch-ups to prevent over-processing.

- Use a light hair oil on your scalp twice a week to keep it moisturised.
- Protect your hair from chlorine and salt damage when you swim by applying an oil-based hair dress or olive oil to your hair before you get into the pool. Shampoo with a clarifying shampoo afterwards.
- Wear a silk or satin scarf or bonnet over your hair when you sleep. Alternatively, use a satin or silk pillow case.

Braids

- Avoid having tightly braided hair as this can result in hair loss.
- Moisturise your scalp daily and cover your hair with a silk-like scarf or bonnet when you sleep.
- Avoid frequent washing of braids as this may lead to frizziness and loosening. Always use a mild shampoo and a leave-in conditioner when you do.
- Avoid using cholesterol-based conditioners.
- Use synthetic hair extensions rather than human hair extensions if you swim frequently.
- After a work out, wipe your scalp with an antiseptic and apply braid spray.

Weaves

- Treat your weave like your own hair. Comb and style it daily.
- Avoid using gels.
- Weaves with glue and adhesives may need more specialist advice so speak with your hairdresser.

References

1. Abii, TA and Amarachi, E. Investigation into the chemical composition of the dry fruit of Tetrapleura tetraptera (Ubikurihu). *Journal of Food Technology* 2007; 5(3): 229-232.
2. Achi, OK. Traditional fermented protein condiments of Nigeria. *African Journal of Biotechnology* 2005; 4(13): 1612-1621.
3. Adebayo-Tayo, BC and Ogunjobi, AA. Comparative effects of oven-drying and sun-drying on the microbiological, proximate nutrient and mineral composition of tympanotonus species (periwinkle) and crassostrea. *Electronic Journal of Environmental Agricultural and Food Chemistry* 2008; 7(4): 2856-2862.
4. Adebayo-Tayo, BC et al. Bacteriological and proximate analysis of periwinkles from two different creeks in Nigeria. *World Applied Sciences Journal* 2006; 1(2): 87-91.
5. Adeboye, AS and Babajide, JM. Effect of processing methods on antinutrients in selected leafy vegetables. *Nigerian Food Journal* 2007; 25(2): 77-87.
6. Adewusi, AG (2004) Potential for the Development and Conservation of Dacroydes edulis in Sakpoba Forest Reserve in Edo state in the Niger Delta area of Nigeria. In: *Forest Products, Livelihood and Conservation - Case Studies in Non-timber Product Systems*, Volume 2, (eds. T. Sunderland and O. Ndoye), The Center for International Forestry Research, Bogor, Indonesia.

7. Adewusi, HA. (1997). The African Star Apple Chrysophyllum albidum: Indigenous Knowledge from Ibadan, south-western Nigeria. In: Proceedings of a National Workshop on the Potential of the Star Apple in Nigeria (eds. O.A Denton, D.O Ladipo, M.A Adetoro, M.B Sarumi), pp 25-33.
8. Agroforestry Tree Database. www.worldagroforestrycentre.org.
9. Agu, HO et al. Quality characteristics of biscuits made from wheat and African breadfruit (Treculia africana). *Nigerian Food Journal* 2007; 25(2): 19-27.
10. Aja, PM et al. Proximate analysis of Talinum triangulare (Water Leaf) leaves and its softening principle. *Pakistan Journal of Nutrition* 2010 (6): 524-526.
11. Akande, M (1979). Bush fowl (Francolin bical carratus) as a pest and potential source of meat in Nigeria. Unpublished thesis. Department of Forestry Resources Management. University of Ibadan, Nigeria.
12. Akinnagbe, A and Oni, O. Quantitative variations in the growth of progeny seedlings of Prosopis africana (Guill., Perrott. and Rich.) plus trees in Nigeria. *African Journal of Biotechnology* 2007; 6(4): 359-363.
13. Akubugwo, IE and Ugbogu, AE. Physicochemical studies on oils from five selected Nigerian plant seeds. *Pakistan Journal of Nutrition* 2007; 6(1): 75-78.
14. Aladesanmi, AJ. Tetrapleura tetraptera: Molluscicidal Activity and chemical constituents. *African Journal of Traditional Complementary and Alternative Medicines* 2007; 4(1): 23 - 36.
15. Amusa, NA et al. Biodeterioration of the African Star Apple (Chrysophyllum albidum) in storage and its effect on its food Value. *African Journal of Biotechnology* 2003; 2(3): 56-59.

16. Asoegwu, S. et al. Physical Properties of African Oil Bean Seed (Pentaclethra macrophylla). *Agricultural Engineering International: the CIGR Ejournal.* Manuscript FP 05 006. Vol. VIII. August, 2006.
17. Baidu-Forson, JJ (1998). Africa's Natural Resources Conservation and Management Surveys - Summary Proceedings of the UNU/INRA Regional Workshop. Accra, Ghana - March 1998. United Nations University Institute for Natural Resources in Africa, Ghana.
18. Barceloux, DG (2008). *Medical Toxicology of Natural Substances: Foods, Fungi, Medicinal Herbs, Plants, and Venomous Animals.* Wiley, New Jersey.
19. Battcock, M and Azam-Ali, S (1998). Fermented Fruits and Vegetables: A Global Perspective. FAO Agricultural Services Bulletin No. 134, Food and Agriculture Organisation of the United Nations, Rome.
20. Bender, D (2005). *A Dictionary of Food and Nutrition.* Oxford University Press, Oxford.
21. Berry, J (1966). *A Dictionary of Sierra Leone Krio.* North Western University, Illinois.
22. Besançon, S. Study of the influence on the glycaemia of different cereals and sauces consumed in Mali. In: Nutritional management of diabetes in Africa: The example of Mali.
23. Besong, M et al (2001). Commercialisation as an incentive and threat for Gnetum species. Paper for presentation at a workshop on the incentive measures for sustainable use and conservation of agrobiodiversity, Lusaka, Zambia, 11-14 September 2001.
24. Bioversity International website. www.bioversityinternational.org.
25. Burkill, HM (1985). *The Useful Plants of West Tropical Africa.* 2nd edition. Volume 1, Families A–D. Royal Botanic Gardens Kew. London

26. Burkill, HM (1994). *The Useful Plants of West Tropical Africa*. 2nd edition. Volume 2, Families E-I. Royal Botanic Gardens Kew. London
27. Burkill, HM (1985). *The Useful Plants of West Tropical Africa*. 2nd edition. Volume 3, Families J-L. Royal Botanic Gardens Kew. London
28. Burkill, HM (1997). *The Useful Plants of West Tropical Africa*. 2nd edition. Volume 4, Families M–R. Royal Botanic Gardens Kew. London
29. Burkill, HM (2000). *The Useful Plants of West Tropical Africa*. 2nd edition. Volume 5, Families S–Z, Addenda. Royal Botanic Gardens Kew. London
30. Cave, B and Coutts, A (2002). Health Evidence Base for the Mayor's Draft Cultural Strategy. http://www.londonshealth.gov.uk/pdf/culture.pdf
31. Centre for Cover Crops Information and Seed Exchange in Africa (2001). Increasing Mucuna's Potential as a Food and Feed Crop. Centre for Cover Crops Information and Seed Exchange in Africa, Benin Republic.
32. Centre for International Forestry Research (1996). Promoting Stewardship of Forests in the Humid Forest Zone of Anglophone West and Central Africa. Centre for International Forestry Research, Bogor Barat, Indonesia.
33. Centre for International Forestry Research. Fact sheet: Njansang (Ricinodendron Heudelotti).
34. Centre for International Forestry Research. Factsheet. Gnetum species (Okok or Eru)
35. Centre for International Forestry Research. Factsheet. Wild mango (Irvingia species).
36. Cobbinah, J (1988). *Snail Farming in West Africa: A practical guide*. Technical Centre for Agriculture and Rural Cooperation, Ede-Wageningen, Netherlands.

37. Consensus Action on Salt and Health. Factsheet: Salt and Black People of African Origin.
38. David, OM and Aderibigbe, EY. Microbiology and proximate composition of 'ogiri', a pastry produced from different melon seeds. *New York Science Journal* 2010; 3(4):18-27.
39. De Foliart, GR (2002).The Human Use of Insects as a Food Resource: A Bibliographic Account in Progress. http://www.food-insects.com/book.
40. De Haas, H (2007). The Myth of Invasion: Irregular Migration from West Africa to the Maghreb and the European Union. International Migration Institute Research Report, James Martin 21st Century School, Oxford University, Oxford.
41. Department of Health (2001). The Health Survey for England – The Health of Minority Ethnic Groups 1999.Department of Health, London.
42. Department of Health (2004). At Least Five a Week: Evidence on the Impact of Physical Activity and its Relationship to Health. Department of Health, London.
43. Department of Health (2008). Healthy Weight, Healthy Lives: Consumer Insight Summary. Department of Health, London.
44. Diabetes UK (2006). Ten steps to eating well for people with diabetes. Diabetes UK, London.
45. Diablo, OK and Behr, T. Processing of mucuna for human food in the Republic of Guinea. *Tropical and Subtropical Agroecosystems* 2003; 1(2-3):193-196.
46. Dike, MC. Proximate, photochemical and nutrient compositions of some fruits, seeds and leaves of some plant species at Mudale, Nigeria. *Journal of Agricultural and Biological Science* 2010; 5(1): 7-16.

47. Dunn-Marcos, R et al (2005). Liberians: An Introduction to their History and Culture. Culture Profile No. 19, (ed. Donald A. Ranard). Centre for Applied Linguistics. Washington DC.
48. Dweck, AC (2001). A Review of Guava (Psidium guajava). http://www.dweckdata.com/Published_papers/Psidium_guajava.pdf.
49. Eddy, NO and Udoh, CL. Proximate evaluation of the nutritional value of some soup thickeners. *ChemClass Journal* 2005, Volume 2(12-14)
50. Edem, DO et al. Chemical evaluation of the nutritive value of the fruit of African Star Apple (Chrysophyllum albidum). *Food Chemistry* 1984; 14(4): 303-311.
51. Edijala, JK. Effects of processing on the thiamin, riboflavin and protein contents of Cowpeas (Vigna unguiculata (L) Walp) II. Alkali ('potash') Treatment. *International Journal of Food Science & Technology* 1980; 15 (4): 445-453.
52. Edmonds, JM and Chwya, J (1997). Black nightshades Solanum nigrum L and related species. International Plant Genetic Resources Institute, Rome.
53. Eleyinmi, AF. Chemical composition and antibacterial activity of Gongronema latifolium. *Journal of Zhejiang University Science B.* 2007; 8(5): 352–358.
54. Essien, EU. Lipid content and fatty acid profiles of some lesser known Nigerian foods. *Journal of Food Biochemistry* 1995; 19(3):153-159.
55. Fagbuaro, O et al. Nutritional status of four species of giant land snails in Nigeria. *Journal of Zhejiang University Science B.* 2006; 7(9):686-689
56. Fandohana, P et al. Fate of aflatoxins and fumonisins during the processing of maize into food products in Benin. *International Journal of Food Microbiology* 2005; 98: 249– 259.

57. Food and Agricultural Organisation of the United Nations. Factsheets for the Pacific.
58. Food and Agriculture Organisation of the United Nations (1989). Utilization of Tropical Foods: Tropical Oil Seeds. Food and Nutrition Paper 47/5. FAO, Rome.
59. Food and Agriculture Organisation of the United Nations (1990). Roots, Tubers, Plantains and Bananas in Human Nutrition. FAO, Rome.
60. Food and Agriculture Organisation of the United Nations (1997). Agriculture, Food and Nutrition for Africa - A Resource Book for Teachers of Agriculture. FAO Rome.
61. Food and Agriculture Organisation of the United Nations (1998). Carbohydrates in Human Nutrition. Report of a Joint FAO/WHO Expert Consultation. FAO Food and Nutrition paper No 66. FAO, Rome.
62. Franco, OH et al. Effects of physical activity on life expectancy with cardiovascular disease. *Archives of Internal Medicine* 2005; 165(20):2355-60.
63. Frison, EA et al (2006). Agricultural biodiversity, nutrition and health: Making a Difference to hunger and nutrition in the developing world. Food and Nutrition Bulletin, 27: 167–179. Consultative Group on International Agricultural Research, Washington DC.
64. Grubben, GJH and Denton, OA (2004). *Vegetables. Plant Resources of Tropical Africa 2.* Plant Resources of Tropical Africa Foundation/Backhuys Publishers/ CTA. Wageningen, Netherlands.
65. Haard, NF et al (1999). Fermented Cereals. A Global perspective. FAO Agricultural Services Bulletin No. 138. FAO, Rome.

66. Health Development Agency (2000). Health Update: Coronary Heart Disease and Stroke. Health Development Agency, London.

67. Health Education Authority (1993). Enjoy Healthy Eating. Health Education Authority, London.

68. Hill, S (1990). *More than Rice and Peas: Guidelines to Improve Food Provision for Black and Ethnic Minorities in Britain*. The Food Commission, London.

69. Holthuis, LB (1980). Shrimps and Prawns of the World. An Annotated Catalogue of Species of Interest to Fisheries, FAO Fisheries Synopsis No. 125, Volume 1. FAO, Rome.

70. Ibe, UO and Orabuike, JC (2009). Production, nutritional, sensory and storage profile of Ogiri from castor oil seed. Briefing paper presented at the DANIDA International Seminar at Ougadougou, Burkina Faso, 16 – 19 February 2009.

71. Ideriah, TJK, Braide, SA and Briggs, AO. Distribution of lead and total hydrocarbon in tissues of periwinkles (Tympanotonus fuscatus and Pachymelania aurita) in the Upper Bonny River. *Nigerian Journal of Applied Sciences & Environmental Management* 2005; 10(2) :145-150

72. Ikediobi, CO. Amino and fatty acid composition of Pentaclethra macrophylla and Treculia africana seeds. *Journal of the American Oil Chemists' Society* 1981; 58(1):30-31.

73. Ikem, RT. A Controlled comparison of the effect of a high fibre diet on the glycaemic and lipid profile of Nigerian clinic patients with Type 2 diabetes. *Pakistan Journal of Nutrition* 2007; 6(2): 111-116.

74. Ikhuoria, EU and Maliki, M. Characterisation of avocado pear (Americana persea) and African pear (Dacroydes edulis) extracts. *African Journal of Biotechnology* 2007; 6(7): 946-948.
75. Jallow, M (1994). Utilisation of Bonga (Ethmalosa fimbriata) in West Africa. Food and Agriculture Organisation of the United Nations, Rome.
76. Jamabo, N and Chinda, A. Aspects of the ecology of Tympanotonus fuscatus var fuscatus (Linnaeus, 1758) in the mangrove swamps of the Upper Bonny River, Niger Delta. *Nigeria Current Research Journal of Biological Sciences* 2010; 2(1): 42-47.
77. Jansen, PCM (2005). Mucuna sloanei Fawc. & Rendle. Record from Protabase. Jansen, P.C.M. & Cardon, D. (Editors). PROTA (Plant Resources of Tropical Africa / Ressources végétales de l'Afrique tropicale), Wageningen, Netherlands.
78. Jenkins, DJA et al. Direct comparison of a dietary portfolio of cholesterol-lowering foods with a statin in hypercholesterolemic participants. *American Journal of Clinical Nutrition* 2005; 81(2):380-387.
79. Joshipura, K et al. Fruit and vegetable intake in relation to risk of ischemic stroke. *Journal of the American Medical Association* 1999; 282: 1233-9.
80. Kant, R. Sweet proteins – Potential replacement for artificial low calorie sweeteners. Review in *Nutrition Journal* 2005; 4:5.
81. Kayode, AAA and Kayode, OT. Some medicinal values of Telfairia occidentalis: A Review. *American Journal of Biochemistry and Molecular Biology* 2011; 1: 30-38.
82. Kittler, PG and Sucher, KP. Accent on Taste: An applied approach to multicultural competency. *Diabetes Spectrum* 17: 200-204, 2004.

83. Kouyaté, AM and van Damme, P (2006). Detarium microcarpum Guill. & Perr. [Internet] Record from Protabase. Schmelzer, G.H. & Gurib-Fakim, A. (Editors). PROTA (Plant Resources of Tropical Africa / Ressources végétales de l'Afrique tropicale), Wageningen, Netherlands.
84. Kraemer, S. The fragile male. *British Medical Journal* 2000; 321: 1609-1612.
85. Malu, SP et al. Analysis of Egeria radiata and Thais coronata shells as an alternative source of calcium for the food industry in Nigeria. *Pakistan Journal of Nutrition* 2009; 8(7): 965-969.
86. Manner, HI (2010). Farm and Forestry Production and Marketing Profile for Tannia (Xanthosoma spp.). In: Elevitch, C.R. (ed.). *Specialty Crops for Pacific Island Agroforestry.* Permanent Agriculture Resources (PAR), Holualoa, Hawaii. http://agroforestry.net/scps.
87. Martin, FW and Ruberte RM (1979). *Edible Leaves of the Tropics*. Antillan College Press, Mayaguez. (3rd Edition) 1998.
88. Martin, RM (1840). *History of the British Colonies*. J Cochrane and Co, London.
89. Mbah, CE and Elekima, GOV. Nutrient composition of some terrestrial insects in Ahmadu Bello University, Samaru Zaria, Nigeria. *Science World Journal* 2007; 2(2):17-20.
90. McLaughlin, J. Plants for use in a traditional African-American yard in Miami-Dade County: Vegetable and fruit crops including a selection of those grown in Africa. University of Florida, Florida. http://miamidade.ifas.ufl.edu/old/programs/urbanhort/publications/PDF/African%20Garden%20vegetable%20and%20fruit.pdf.

91. McRae, TE and Paul, AA (1979). *Foods of Rural Gambia*. Medical Research Council Dunn Nutrition Centre, Cambridge UK and Keneba, The Gambia. (2nd edition) 1996.

92. Mialoundama, F (1993). Nutritional and Socio-economic Value of Gnetum Leaves in Central African Forest. In Hladik, C. M. et al., *Tropical Forest, People and Food: Biocultural Interactions and Applications to Development*. Parthenon Publishing Group, Carnforth, UK.

93. Ministry of Agriculture Fisheries and Foods (1995). *Manual of Nutrition*. HMSO, London.

94. Molin, G. Probiotics in foods not containing milk or milk constituents, with special reference to Lactobacillus plantarum 299v Supplement in *American Journal of Clinical Nutrition* 2001; 73(2): 380S-385s.

95. MORI (2005). High Blood Pressure in Lambeth and Southwark. Market & Opinion Research International, Ltd

96. National Institute for Health and Clinical Excellence. Opportunities for and barriers to good nutritional health in minority ethnic groups.

97. National Research Council (1996). *Lost Crops of Africa Volume I: Grains*. National Academy Press, Washington DC.

98. National Research Council (2006). *Lost Crops of Africa Volume II: Vegetables*. National Academy Press, Washington DC.

99. National Research Council (2008). *Lost Crops of Africa Volume III: Fruits*. National Academy Press, Washington DC.

100. Ndem, JI, Akpanabiatu MI and Essien EU. Effect of seafood (Periwinkle, Bonga fish and Crayfish) and vegetable oil-enriched meals on cardiovascular disease. *Pakistan Journal of Nutrition* 2008; 7(4): 603-606.

101. Njoku, HO., Eli, I and Ofuya, CO. Effect of pre-treatment on the cooking time of the African Yam Bean (Sphenostylis sternocarpa). *Journal of Food Science* 1989; 54(3):758-759.

102. Nutrition Sub-committee of the Diabetes Care Advisory Committee of Diabetes UK. The dietitians challenge: the implementation of nutritional advice for people with diabetes. *Journal of Human Nutrition and Dietetics* 2003; 16(1): 421-152.

103. Nyunaï, N (2008). Beilschmiedia mannii (Meisn.) Benth. & Hook.f. [Internet] Record from Protabase. Louppe, D., Oteng-Amoako, A.A. & Brink, M. (Editors). PROTA (Plant Resources of Tropical Africa / Ressources végétales de l'Afrique tropicale), Wageningen, Netherlands

104. O'Connor, CB. (1993). *Traditional Cheese-making Manual.* ILCA (International Livestock Centre for Africa), Addis Ababa, Ethiopia.

105. Oboh, FOJ and Masodje, HI. Nutritional and antimicrobial properties of Vernonia amygdalina Leaves. *International Journal of Biomedical and Health Sciences* 2009; 5(2): 51-56.

106. Oboh, G and Akindahunsi, AA. Change in the ascorbic acid, total phenol and antioxidant activity of sun-dried commonly consumed green leafy vegetables in Nigeria. *Nutrition and Health.* 2004; 18(1):29-36.

107. Odebunmi, EO et al. Proximate and nutritional composition of Kola nut (Cola nitida), Bitter cola (Garcinia cola) and Alligator pepper (Afromomum melegueta). Short Communication in *African Journal of Biotechnology* 2009; 8(2): 308-310.

108. Odenigbo, UM and Obizoba, IC. Effects of food processing techniques on the nutrient and anti-nutrient composition of Afzelia africana (Akparata). *Journal of Biomedical Investigation* 2004: 2(2):86-91.

109. Odugbemi T (2006). *Outlines and Pictures of Medicinal Plants from Nigeria*, 1st edition. University of Lagos Press, Lagos.
110. Odukoya, OA et al. Antioxidant activity of Nigerian dietary spices. *Electronic Journal of Environmental Agriculture and Food Chemistry* 2005; 4(6): 1086-1093.
111. Ogunshe, AAO, Omotosho, MO and Ayansina, ADV. Microbial studies and biochemical characteristics of controlled fermented Afiyo - a Nigerian fermented food condiment from Prosopis africana (Guill and Perr.) Taub. *Pakistan Journal of Nutrition* 2007; 6(6): 620-627.
112. Ojekale, AB., Makinde, SCO and Osileye, O. Phytochemistry and antimicrobial evaluation of Thaumatococcus danielli, Benn. (Benth.) leaves. *Nigerian Food Journal* 2007; 25(2):176-183.
113. Okafor, JC (1999). The Use of Farmer Knowledge in Non-wood Forest Product Research. In: *Current Research Issues and Prospects for Conservation and Development.* FAO, Rome.
114. Okafor, JC. Conservation and use of traditional vegetables from woody forest species in south-eastern Nigeria. In Traditional African Vegetables. Proceedings of the IPGRI International Workshop on Genetic Resources of Traditional Vegetables in Africa: Conservation and Use (ed. L. Guarino). ICRAF-HQ, Nairobi, Kenya, 29-31 August 1995.
115. Okigbo, BN (1980). Nutritional Implications of Projects Giving High Priority to the Production of Staples of Low Nutritive Quality: The Case for Cassava (Manihot esculenta, Crantz) in the Humid Tropics of West Africa. International Institute of Tropical Agriculture, Ibadan, Nigeria.
116. Okorie, HA et al. Studies on pomology of the African pear (Dacryodes edulis (G. Don) HJ Lam) in Nigeria. *Acta Horticulturae* (ISHS) 2000; 531: 207-212.

117. Okwu, DU and Ibeawuchi, CU. Nutritive value of Monodora myristica and Xylopia aethiopica as additives in traditional foodstuffs. *Journal of Medicinal and Aromatic Plant Sciences* 2005; 27, 275-279.

118. Olapade, A and Adetuyi, DO. Comparison of different methods of producing bambara (Voandzeia subterranean L. Thou) flours for preparation of 'moin-moin'. *Nigerian Food Journal* 2007; 25(2): 150-157.

119. Oluba, AM et al. Fatty acid composition of Citrullus lanatus (Egusi melon) oil and its effect on serum lipids and some serum enzymes. *The Internet Journal of Cardiovascular Research* (5):2.

120. Omafuvbe, BO et al. Chemical and biochemical changes in African locust bean and melon during fermentation to condiments. *Pakistan Journal of Nutrition* 2004; 3(3): 140-145.

121. Onyechi, UA, Judd PA, and Ellis PR. African plant foods rich in non-starch polysaccharides reduce postprandial blood glucose and insulin concentrations in healthy human subjects. *British Journal of Nutrition* 1998; 80(5):419-28.

122. Onweluzo, J and Eilitta, M. Surveying Mucuna utilisation as a food in Enugu and Kogi states of Nigeria. *Tropical and Subtropical Agroecosystems* 2003; 1(2-3):213-225.

123, O'Reilly-Wright, E (1964). *The Student's Cookery Book*. Oxford University Press, Oxford.

124. Osseo-Asare, F (2005). *Food Culture in Sub-Saharan Africa*. Greenwood Press, Westport, CT.

125. Oyeowo, EO (1988). Tolerance tests with three refined petroleum products and an edible mollusc Tympanotonus fuscauta (linne). Nigerian Institute for Oceanography and Marine Research, Lagos.

126. Palada, MC and Crossman, SMA (1999). Evaluation of Tropical Leaf Vegetables in the Virgin Islands. p. 388–393. In: J. Janick (ed.), *Perspectives on New Crops and New Uses*. ASHS Press, Alexandria, VA.

127. Parkouda C., Diawara, B and Ouoba, LII. Technology and physico-chemical characteristics of Bikalga, alkaline fermented seeds of Hibiscus sabdariffa. *African Journal of Biotechnology* 2008; 7(7): 916-922.

128. Peace Corps Sierra Leone (1985). *Krio language Manual*. Peace Corps Sierra Leone.

129. Plenderleith, K (2000). Ricinodendron Heudelotti: A State of Knowledge Study undertaken for the Central African Regional Program for the Environment. Oxford Forestry Institute Department of Plant Sciences, University of Oxford, United Kingdom.

130. Quattrocchi, U (1999). *CRC World Dictionary of Plant Names: Common Names, Scientific Names, Eponyms, Synonyms, and Etymology*. CRC Press, Florida.

131. Raheem, B (2006). Developments and microbiological applications in African foods: Emphasis on Nigerian wara cheese. Academic dissertation. University of Helsinki, Finland.

132. Reid, DG et al. Mudwhelks and mangroves: The evolutionary history of an ecological association (Gastropoda: Potamididae) *Molecular Phylogenetics and Evolution* 2008; 47: 680–699.

133. Rolls, BJ et al. Portion size of food affects energy intake in normal-weight and overweight men and women. *American Journal of Clinical Nutrition* 2002; 76(6): 1207-1213.

134. Salem, ML. Dietary supplementation with Cyperus esculentus L (Tiger nut) tubers attenuated atherosclerotic lesion in apolipoprotein E knockout mouse

associated with inhibition of inflammatory cell responses. *American Journal of Immunology* 2005; 1(1): 60-67.

135. Seidemann, J (2005). *World Spice Plants: Economic Usage, Botany, Taxonomy* (4th edition). Springer, New York.
136. Shackleton, CM, Pasquini, M and Drescher, AW (2009). *African Indigenous Vegetables in Urban Agriculture*. Earthscan, London.
137. Solomons, NW. Diet and Long Term Health: An African Diaspora Perspective. *Asia Pacific Journal of Clinical Nutrition* 2003; 12:313–330.
138. Steinkraus, KH (1996). *Handbook of Indigenous Fermented Food.* CRC Press, Florida.
139. Stumpf, E (1998). Post-harvest loss due to pests in dried cassava chips and comparative methods for its assessment - A case study on small-scale farm households in Ghana. FAO, Rome.
140. Tchoundjeu, Z and Atangana, AR (2006). Fruits for the future 7. Ndjanssang Ricinodendron heudelotii (Baill.). Southampton Centre for Underutilised Crops, University of Southampton, Southampton.
141. Tekwe, C., Ndam, N and Nkefor, JP (2003). Gnetum domestication for livelihood improvement and conservation. Paper submitted to the 12th World Forestry Congress, Quebec City, Canada, 2003.
142. The American Dietetic Association (2007). Position paper: Total diet approach to communicating food and nutrition information. In *Journal of the American Dietetic Association* 2007:1224 –1232.
143. The International Institute of Tropical Agriculture. Banana and Plantain Systems program. http://www.iita.org/web/iita/programs/banana-and-plaintain-systems.

144. The International Institute of Tropical Agriculture. The Integrated Cassava Project. www.cassavabiz.org.

145. Tropical Plant Walk at The African Pavilion 2009. http://www.nczoo.org/animals/Africa/NCZoo_TropPlantWalk09.pdf.

146. Tubene, SL (2004). *Ethnic and Speciality Vegetables Handbook*, 1st edition. University of Maryland, Maryland.

147. Tudor-Locke, C (2002). Taking Steps toward Increased Physical Activity: Using Pedometers to Measure and Motivate. President's Council on Physical Fitness and Sports Research Digest, Series 3 number 17.

148. Udofia, US. Snail (Archachatina marginata) pie: A nutrient rich snack for school-age children and young mothers. *International Journal of Food Safety, Nutrition and Public Health* 2009; 2(2):125 - 130.

149. Westphal-Stevels, JMC (1986). Local vegetables in Cameroon: Corchorus species used as a vegetable. In: First international symposium on taxonomy of cultivated plants. Acta-Horticulturae No.182, pp.423-5. ISHS, Wageningen (Netherlands).

150. Wokoma, EC and Aziagba, GCJ. Sensory evaluation of dawadawa produced by the traditional fermentation of African Yam Bean (Sphenostylis Steno-carpa Harms) Seeds. *Journal of Applied Sciences and Environmental Management* 2001; 5(1):85-91.

151. World Cancer Research Fund (2007). Food, Nutrition, Physical activity and the prevention of cancer: A Global perspective. Recommendations for cancer prevention. World Cancer Research Fund, London.

152. World Health Organisation (2002). The World Health Report 2002 - Reducing Risks, Promoting Healthy Life. World Health Organisation, Geneva.

Index

F

G

H

I

Also available from the same author:

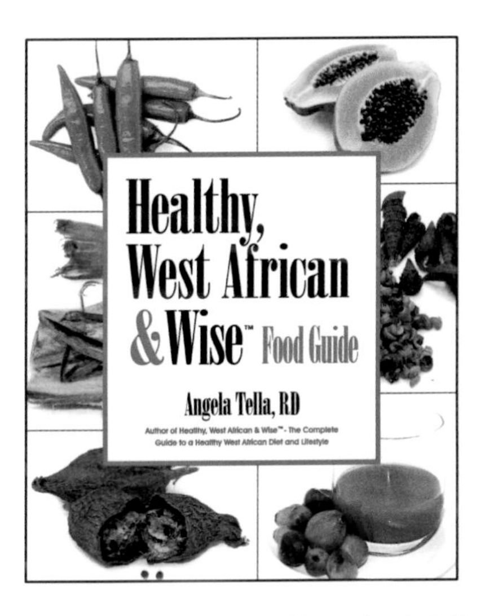

How much do you know about West African foods? If you enjoy West African food and have ever wondered about its nutritional benefits then the *Healthy, West African & Wise™ Food Guide* is the book you've been waiting for.

With colour pictures and profiling 80 foods that feature in the West African diet, this unique book provides invaluable nutritional information and highlights fascinating facts about each food and its use in West African cuisine.

Written as a companion to *Healthy, West African & Wise™ Complete Guide to a Healthy West African Diet and Lifestyle*, this food guide is a must-read, empowering you to eat better today for a healthier tomorrow.